TABLE OF CONTENTS

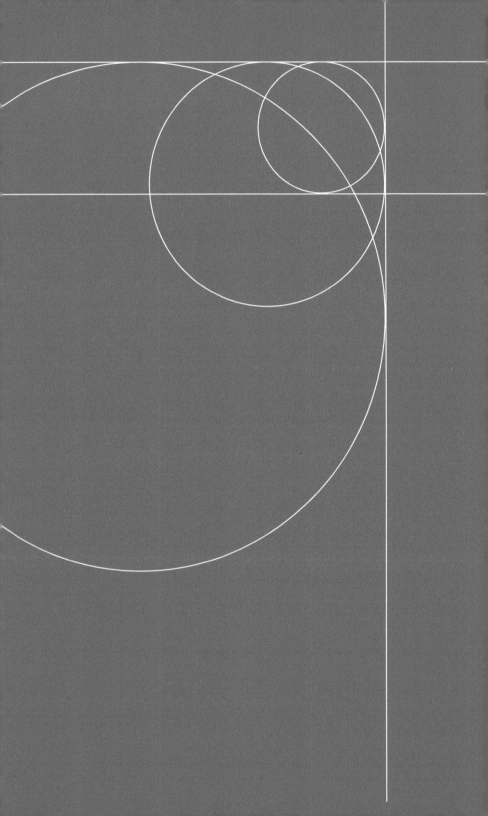

The
Pocket Primer on the Rheumatic Diseases
Second Edition

John H. Klippel, MD, Editor

John H. Stone, MD, MPH, Associate Editor
Leslie J. Crofford, MD, Associate Editor
Patience H. White, MD, MA, Associate Editor

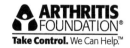

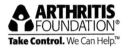

ISBN 978-1-84882-855-1

© Springer-Verlag London Limited 2010

First edition published in 2003 by the Arthritis Foundation, Atlanta, Georgia, USA (ISBN 978-0-912423-38-8)

Apart from any fair dealing for the purposes of research or private study, or criticism or review, as permitted under the Copyright, Designs and Patents Act 1988, this publication may only be reproduced, stored or transmitted, in any form or by any means, with the prior permission in writing of the publishers, or in the case of reprographic reproduction in accordance with the terms of licenses issued by the Copyright Licensing Agency. Enquiries concerning reproduction outside those terms should be sent to the publishers.

The use of registered names, trademarks, etc., in this publication does not imply, even in the absence of a specific statement, that such names are exempt from the relevant laws and regulations and therefore free for general use.

Product liability: The publisher can give no guarantee for information about drug dosage and application thereof contained in this book. In every individual case the respective user must check its accuracy by consulting other pharmaceutical literature.

Printed on acid-free paper

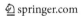 springer.com

The content of the book and the opinions reflected in the text are those of the contributing authors and editors and, therefore, do not necessarily reflect the opinions of the publisher or sponsor.

Many thanks to Dr. John Stone for lending his expertise and hard work in developing and editing this work.

CONTRIBUTORS

The following people contributed to the *Primer on the Rheumatic Diseases* by writing or revising chapters and sections for the publication of the thirteenth edition. Credits for illustrations are given in figure legends.

Roy D. Altman, MD

Erin L. Arnold, MD

William J. Arnold, MD

Alan N. Baer, MD

W. Timothy Ballard, MD

Joan M. Bathon, MD

Thomas D. Beardmore, MD, FACP, FACR

Francis Berenbaum, MD, PhD

Joseph J. Biundo, Jr., MD

Linda K. Bockensted, MD

David Borenstein, MD

Teresa J. Brady, PhD

Juergen Braun, MD

Maya H. Buch, MBchB, MRCP

Joseph A. Buckwalter, MS, MD

Gerd-Rüdiger Burmester, MD

Frank Buttgereit, MD

Jill P. Buyon, MD

Leonard H. Calabrese, DO

Kenneth T. Calamia, MD

Jeffrey P. Callen, MD

Juan J. Canoso, MD, FACP, MACR

Rowland W. Chang, MD, MPH

Edward S. Chen, MD

Lan X. Chen, MD, PhD

Hyon K. Choi, MD, MPH, DrPH, FRCPC

Daniel J. Clauw, MD

Andrew J. Cooper, MD

Leslie J. Crofford, MD

Dina Dadabhoy, MD

Troy Daniels, DDS, MS

John C. Davis, Jr., MD, MPH

William J. Didie, MD

Paul Dieppe, MD

N. Lawrence Edwards, MD

Hani S. El-Gabalawy, MD, FRCPC

Kevin Elias, MD

John M. Esdaile, MD, MPH

Adel G. Fam, MD, FRCP(C), FACP

Laura M. Fayad, MD

Gary S. Firestein, MD

Kenneth H. Fye, MD

Dafna D. Gladman, MD, FRCPC

Duncan A. Gordon, MD, FRCPC, MACR

Jörg J. Goronzy, MD

Philip J. Hashkes, MD, MSc

George Ho Jr., MD

William A. Horton, MD

Robert D. Inman, MD

Preeti Jaggi, MD

Amy H. Kao, MD, MPH

Daniel L. Kastner, MD, PhD

Jonathan Kay, MD

James Kelley, PhD

Robert P. Kimberly, MD

CONTRIBUTORS (continued)

John H. Klippel, MD

Denise Kruszewski, MS

Ronald M. Laxer, MD, FRCPC

Carol B. Lindsley, MD

Geoffrey Littlejohn, MD, MPH, MBBS[Hon], FRACP, FRCP(Edin)

Daniel J. Lovell, MD, MPH

Harvinder S. Luthra, MD

Susan Manzi, MD, MPH

David Marker, BS

Manuel Martinez-Lavin, MD

Maureen D. Mayes, MD, MPH

Geraldine McCarthy, MD, FRCPI

Philip J. Mease, MD

Peter A. Merkel, MD, MPH

Frederick W. Miller, MD, PhD

Michael A. Mont, MD

Kerstin Morehead, MD

Barry L. Myones, MD

Chester V. Oddis, MD

Alyce M. Oliver, MD, PhD

John J. O'Shea, MD

Michelle Petri, MD, MPH

David S. Pisetsky, MD, PhD

Reed Edwin Pyeritz, MD, PhD

James D. Reeves, MD

Lisa G. Rider, MD

Christopher Ritchlin, MD

David B. Robinson, MD, MSc, FRCPC

Ann K. Rosenthal, MD

Keith T. Rott, MD, PhD

John G. Ryan, MB, MRCPI

Kenneth G. Saag, MD, MSc

Carlo Salvarani, MD

Philip Sambrook, MD, FRACP

Pasha Sarraf, MD, PhD

H. Ralph Schumacher, MD

William W. Scott, Jr., MD

Sean P. Scully, MD, PhD

James R. Seibold, MD

Philip Seo, MD, MHS

Thorsten M. Seyler, MD

Leena Sharma, MD

Stanford Shulman, MD

Richard Siegel, MD, PhD

Robert F. Spiera, MD

E. William St. Clair, MD

John H. Stone, MD, MPH

Christopher V. Tehlirian, MD

Robert A. Terkeltaub, MD

Désirée Van der Heijde, MD, PhD

John Varga, MD

Jean-Marc Waldenburger, MD, PhD

Nelson B. Watts, MD

Sterling West, MD

Cornelia M. Weyand, MD

Patience H. White, MD, MA

John B. Winfield, MD

Patricia Woo, BSc, MBBS, PhD, MRCP, FRCP, CBE

Robert L. Wortmann, MD, FACP, FACR

Steven R. Ytterberg, MD

Alex Zautra, PhD

INTRODUCTION

For eight decades the *Primer on the Rheumatic Diseases* has been the standard text from which most medical students and house officers have learned rheumatology. I myself will never forget thumbing through an older edition of the *Primer* as a second-year resident, while waiting to review a perplexing patient with my tutor. Fortunately the tutor was running late with his own patients, so I had time to flip through the book – then much thinner – a couple of times. While turning the pages, perusing the features of those diseases whose names were still exotic to me, and considering my patient's history of conductive hearing loss and pulmonary nodules, a light went on when I stumbled eventually on a particular chapter. I still remember the jaw-dropping effect on my tutor of my announcement then that I had a patient with Wegener's granulomatosis. I think I became a rheumatologist that very moment!

Subsequent editions of the *Primer* have suffered from the inevitable "obesity creep," making it an outstanding reference textbook but virtually impossible to flip through quickly while awaiting one's tutor, and even more difficult to slip into the pocket of a white coat to carry on rounds. For this reason we have created the *Pocket Primer*, a mini version that cuts the larger book down to its essentials. Each chapter contains succinct descriptions of the diagnostic approach to and clinical manifestations, laboratory features, and strategies for the management and therapy of a particular rheumatic disease.

In editing the second edition of this book I am delighted to note the updating which has had to occur, not only of the first edition of the *Pocket Primer* but also of the more recent thirteenth edition of the larger *Primer on the Rheumatic Diseases*. The field of rheumatology remains lively, progressive, and fascinating to all who love the practice of medicine, regardless of specialty. Tutors, trainees, and practitioners will all find the *Pocket Primer* a handy guide to the rheumatic diseases and a superb overview of the latest advances in treatment.

JOHN H. STONE, MD, MPH
Director of Clinical Rheumatology
Massachusetts General Hospital

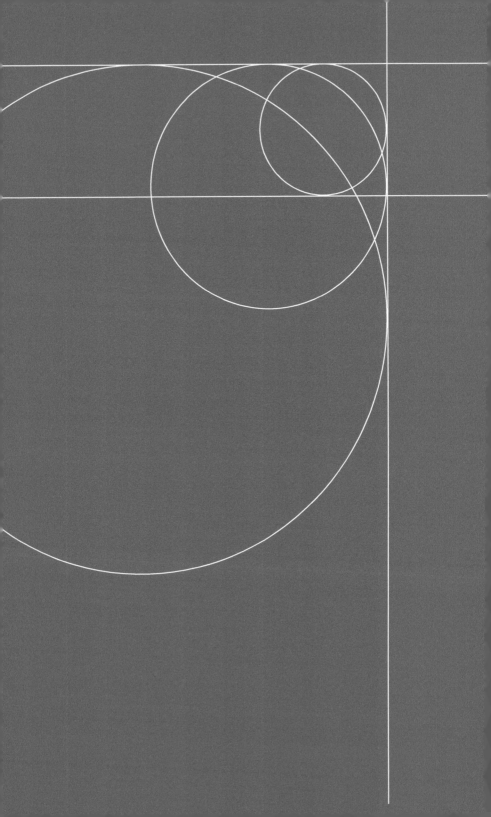

1 HISTORY AND PHYSICAL EXAMINATION

Conducting a careful history and physical examination to determine the onset and course of signs and symptoms, functional impairments caused by the arthritis, and the presence or absence of pathology or dysfunction in musculoskeletal structures is essential.

History

A thoughtful, detailed history is critical in determining the nature of the complaint and helps focus the clinical exam. Structure the history to answer these questions.

- Is the problem regional or generalized, symmetric or asymmetric, peripheral or central? Is it acute, subacute, or chronic? Is it progressive?

- Do the symptoms suggest inflammation or damage to musculoskeletal structures?

- Is there evidence of a systemic process? Are there associated extra-articular features?

- Has there been functional loss and disability?

- Is there a family history of a similar or related problem?

GALS (Gait, Arms, Legs, Spine) Screening

By asking three basic questions and systematically examining the patient's gait, arms, legs, and spine, the physician can rapidly screen for musculoskeletal disease.

- Have you any pain or stiffness in your muscles, joints, or back?

- Can you dress yourself completely without any difficulty?

- Can you walk up and down stairs without any difficulty?

Main Features of the Gait, Arms, Legs, Spine (GALS) Screening Inspection

Position/activity	Normal findings
Gait	Symmetry, smoothness of movement Normal stride length Normal heel strike, stance, toe-off, swing-through Able to turn quickly
Inspection from behind	Straight spine Normal, symmetric paraspinal muscles Normal shoulder and gluteal muscle bulk Level iliac crests No popliteal cysts No popliteal swelling No hindfoot swelling/deformity
Inspection from the side	Normal cervical and lumbar lordosis Normal thoracic kyphosis
"Touch your toes"	Normal lumbar spine (and hip) flexion
Inspection from the front Arms "Place your hands behind your head (elbows out)"	Normal glenohumeral, sternoclavicular, and acromioclavicular joint movement
"Place your hands by your side (elbows straight)"	Full elbow extension
"Place your hands in front (palms down)"	No wrist/finger swelling or deformity Able to fully extend fingers
"Turn your hands over"	Normal supination/pronation Normal palms
"Make a fist"	Normal grip power
"Place the tip of each finger on the tip of the thumb"	Normal fine precision, pinch
Legs	Normal quadriceps bulk/symmetry No knee swelling or deformity No forefoot/midfoot deformity Normal arches No abnormal callus formation
Spine "Place your ear on your shoulder"	Normal cervical lateral flexion

Reproduced from Doherty M, Dacre J, Dieppe P, Snaith M. The GALS locomotor screen. Ann Rheum Dis 1992; 51: 1165–1169. Copyright © 1992 BMJ Publishing Group Ltd, with permission from BMJ Publishing Group Ltd.

Examination of Specific Joint Areas

Any abnormalities detected through the GALS screening are followed with a more detailed examination.

Hand and Wrist

- **Alignment** – Inspect alignment of the digits relative to the wrist and forearm.

- **Nails** – Inspect nails for evidence of onycholysis or pitting suggestive of psoriasis. Inspect nail fold capillaries for redness and telangiectasia, indicative of a connective-tissue disease.

- **Skin** – Look for tightening of the skin around the digits, or sclerodactyly, typical of scleroderma.

- **Finger joints** – Inspect and palpate distal interphalangeal (DIP) and proximal interphalangeal (PIP) joints for swelling, which may signify bony osteophytes, synovitis, or an intra-articular effusion. Look for fullness in the valleys normally found between the knuckles (heads of the metacarpal bones), indicating swelling of the metacarpophalangeal (MCP) joints. Palpate individual hand joints to determine the presence of joint-line tenderness and effusion, important indicators of synovitis.

- **Palms** – Inspect the palmar aspect of the hands to identify atrophy of the thenar or hypothenar eminences, which can result from disuse due to articular involvement of the fingers or wrists or, in the case of the thenar eminence, carpal tunnel syndrome.

- **Wrist**

  - **Dorsum** – Note swelling on the dorsum of the wrist. Have patient gently wiggle the fingers to differentiate between synovitis of the wrist and tenosynovitis of the extensor tendons. Swelling tends to move with the tendons if it is a result of tenosynovitis. Palpate the dorsum of the joint to detect synovial thickening and tenderness suggestive of wrist joint synovitis.

  - **Ulnar styloid** – Check for swelling and tenderness in the area just distal to the ulnar styloid, where the extensor and flexor carpi ulnaris tendons are directly palpable. This area is commonly involved in early RA.

— **Radial aspect** – Evaluate pain and tenderness confined to the radial aspect of the wrist, which are due most commonly to OA of the first carpometacarpal joint or to DeQuervain's tenosynovitis.

— **Function** – Evaluate global function of the hand by asking the patient to make a fist, and then fully extend and spread out the digits. Test pincer function of the thumb and fingers. Estimate grip strength by having the patient squeeze two of the examiner's fingers.

Elbow

● **Anatomy** – Identify the olecranon process, the medical and lateral epicondyles of the humerus, and the radial head. Locate the triangular recess formed in the lateral aspect of the joint between the olecranon process, in the lateral epicondyle, and the radial head. This recess is the point where the synovial cavity of the elbow is most accessible to inspection and palpation.

● **Bulging** – Look for bulging in this triangular recess to identify an effusion and synovitis. In contrast, swelling directly over the olecranon process is more suggestive of olecranon bursitis.

● **Contracture** – Have the patient extend the forearm as much as possible to detect the presence of a flexion contracture, an almost invariant feature of elbow synovitis.

● **Tennis elbow** – Palpate the lateral epicondyle for tenderness, suggesting lateral epicondylitis.

Shoulder

● **Observe** – Examine visually the entire shoulder girdle area, from the front and the back. Note shoulder height. Patients with rotator cuff tears often hold the affected shoulder higher than the other side.

- **Osteophytes** – Look for a prominent bump in the area of the acromioclavicular joint, often associated with osteophytes resulting from OA.

- **Atrophy** – Look for atrophy of the shoulder girdle musculature, an important sign of chronic glenohumeral joint pathology, as occurs in RA.

- **Effusion**s – Look for effusions in the shoulder joint, which are visible anteriorly just medial to the area of the bicipital groove and, if large enough, also are evident laterally below the acromion.

- **Motion** – Have the patient demonstrate active range of motion of the arms in several planes. Internal and external rotations of the shoulder are particularly sensitive to glenohumeral pathology. Test passive range of motion, particularly internal/external rotation and abduction.

- **Palpate** – Palpate the entire shoulder girdle, the cervical spine, and the thoracic wall.

Hip

- **Groin pain** – Pain in the groin (or less commonly the buttock) that tends to radiate down the anteromedial aspect of the thigh is often a result of hip arthritis.

- **Trochanteric pain** – Pain in the lateral trochanteric area is most often indicative of bursitis involving the trochanteric bursa.

- **Gait** – Note a "coxalgic" gait, quickly swinging the pelvis forward on the affected side to avoid weight-bearing on the affected hip, an indication of true hip disease.

- **Motion** – Test hip range of motion by having the patient actively flex, extend, abduct, and abduct the leg. Screen passive range of motion with the patient supine and "log rolling" the entire extended leg. The leg then is flexed maximally to assess completeness of this motion.

- **Internal rotation** – Note pain and loss of motion on internal rotation, particularly sensitive indicators of hip pathology.

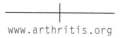

Sacroiliac Joint

- **Palpate joint** – Palpate the sacroiliac (SI) joint with the patient lying flat on the abdomen. Find the SI joint by placing the palm of the examiner's hand around the iliac crest; the thumb tends to fall directly over the joint. Apply direct pressure with the thumb in this area to elicit tenderness in the SI joint.

- **Palpate sacrum** – Apply direct pressure over the sacrum to elicit pain in an inflamed SI joint.

- **Gaenslen's maneuver** – Perform Gaenslen's maneuver by having the patient hyperextend the leg over the edge of the examining table, thereby stressing the ipsilateral SI joint.

Spine

- **Observe** – Examine the spine initially with the patient standing and the entire spine visible. Evaluate the normal curvature of the spine, lumbar lordosis, thoracic kyphosis, and cervical lordosis by observing the patient from the back and the side, and noting any loss or accentuation of these curves.

- **Scoliosis** – Observe true scoliosis irrespective of the state of spinal flexion. A functional scoliosis due to leg-length discrepancy decreases with spinal flexion.

- **Motion** – Examine the range of motion of the entire spine in segments.

- **Lumbar** – The Schober test (movement of a 10-cm segment from the lumbosacral junction with spine flexion) is performed to specifically assess movement in the lumbar spine.

- **Lumbosacral** – Examine the lumbosacral area and perform a detailed neurologic examination of the leg in patients presenting with symptoms suggestive of a lumbar radiculopathy, such as pain and paresthesia shooting down the leg.

- **Thoracic** – Examine thoracic motion by measuring chest expansion at the level of the nipples. Ankylosing spondylitis can markedly reduce chest expansion from the normal 5–6 cm.

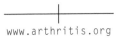

- **Cervical** – Test cervical range of motion with the patient upright and while lying down. Flex, extend, laterally flex (patient attempts to touch the ear to the shoulder), and laterally rotate (patient attempts to touch the chin to the shoulder) the head.

Knee

- **Observe** – Inspect the knee from both the front and the back, with the patient standing.

- **Atrophy** – Atrophy of the quadriceps usually indicates chronic knee pathology.

- **Suprapatellar bursa** – Inspect suprapatellar bursa for evidence of swelling due to synovial-fluid accumulation or synovial infiltration and thickening.

- **Varus deformities** – Varus deformities cause a bow-legged appearance, resulting most commonly from OA preferentially involving the medial compartment.

- **Valgus deformities** – Valgus deformities cause a knock-kneed appearance, more commonly associated with RA.

- **Palpate** – Palpate for tenderness the medial and lateral joint line with the patient lying supine and the knee in partial flexion.

- **Suprapatellar distension** – Distension of the joint in the suprapatellar area and in the medial and lateral compartments indicates large amounts of synovial fluid in the knee.

- **Ligaments** – Test the medial and collateral ligaments by gently applying varus and valgus stresses to the joint while the examiner firmly supports the joint with one hand or immobilizes the joint. Test the cruciate ligaments by using the drawer sign, in which anteroposterior stress is placed on the upper tibia with the knee in flexion; instability of the ligaments will result in the tibia moving back and forth relative to the femur.

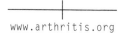

Ankle and Hindfoot

- **Observe** – Examine the ankle and hindfoot as a unit.

- **Valgus deformities** – Detect valgus deformities of the ankle and hindfoot by inspecting the area from behind, with the patient standing.

- **Palpate** – Palpate the joint line of the ankle anteriorly. Boggy swelling and tenderness in this area are typical of ankle synovitis.

- **Achilles tendon** – Look for tenderness and swelling posteriorly, at the insertion of the Achilles tendon, usually indicating enthesitis.

- **Heel** – Look for tenderness in the heel, indicating plantar fasciitis, another enthesitis associated with spondyloarthropathies.

- **Talotibial joint** – Test for ankle synovitis by eliciting pain and limitation in the talotibial joint, capable only of dorsal and plantar flexion.

- **Subtalar joint** – Test the subtalar joint by rocking the calcaneus from side to side while holding the talus stable.

Midfoot and Forefoot

- **Arches** – Note pes planus (flat foot, collapsed arch) or pes cavus (high arch) with the patient standing.

- **Bunions** – Look for hallux valgus deformities, which cause bunions.

- **Daylight sign** – Observe a visible spreading of the toes caused by swelling of the metatarsophalangeal (MTP) joints.

- **Hammertoe** – Observe hammertoe deformity, which in cases of advanced RA results from the subluxation of the MTP joint.

- **Interphalangeal joints** – Observe inflammation of the interphalangeal joints of the toes, common with spondyloarthropathies.

- **Calluses** – Calluses tend to occur in conjunction with subluxation of the MTP joint, where the metatarsal head can be directly palpated subcutaneously.

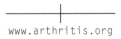

2 LABORATORY ASSESSMENT

Laboratory tests can help confirm a diagnosis suggested by history and physical examination, but are not diagnostic on their own. In addition, laboratory tests can help monitor disease activity, but are meaningful only when they correlate with clinical findings.

Acute-Phase Reactants
Erythrocyte Sedimentation Rate (ESR)

Values

- **Normal for women** – ≤15 mm/h.

- **Normal for men** – ≤10 mm/h.

- **Adjust values** – Adjust normal values for age of patient. Upper limit for men = age divided by 2. Upper limit for women = age plus 10, divided by 2.

Interpretation

- **Elevated** – An elevated ESR reflects active inflammation and is used to determine or monitor disease activity in inflammatory and autoimmune forms of arthritis. Elevations of ESR may also be seen with infections and neoplastic diseases.

- **Factors that increase** – ESR increases with anemia, renal failure, hypergammaglobulinemia, and pregnancy.

- **Factors that decrease** – ESR decreases with changes in red blood cell morphology, hypofibrinogenemia, cryoglobulinemia, and congestive heart failure.

C-Reactive Protein

Values

- **Normal** – <1.0 mg/dl.

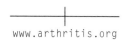

Interpretation

- **Elevated** – An elevated CRP reflects active inflammation and may be used to determine or monitor disease activity in inflammatory or autoimmune forms of arthritis.

- **Normal** – A normal CRP level does not necessarily indicate absence of inflammation.

- **Rapid changes** – CRP levels change rapidly after tissue injury, making this test a more timely indicator of disease activity than ESR.

Rheumatoid Factor

Values

- **Positive** – >1/20 by latex fixation method or ≥20 IU by nephelometry.

Interpretation

- **Healthy people** – 1–2% of healthy people have detectable serum RF; increases with age.

- **RA** – 75% of people with RA have positive RF ("seropositive RA").

Selected Diseases Associated with Elevated Serum Rheumatoid Factors

Chronic bacterial infections	**Parasitic diseases**
Subacute bacterial endocarditis	
Leprosy	**Chronic inflammatory disease of uncertain etiology**
Tuberculosis	
Syphilis	Sarcoidosis
Lyme disease	Periodontal disease
	Pulmonary interstitial disease
	Liver disease
Viral diseases	
Rubella	
Cytomegalovirus	**Mixed cryoglobulinemia**
Infectious mononucleosis	
Influenza	**Hypergammaglobulinemic purpura**

Modified from Koopman WJ, Schrohenber RE. Rheumatoid factor. In: Utsinger PD, Zvaifler MJ, Ehrlich GE (eds). Rheumatoid Arthritis: Etiology, Diagnosis and Therapy. Philadelphia, PA: JB Lippincott, 1985; pp 217–241.

Antinuclear Antibody (ANA)

Values

- **Positive** – >1/40. Many healthy individuals have low titers of ANA. The higher the ANA titer the greater the likelihood that it is associated with an autoimmune condition. However, in all cases, serological findings such as ANA assays require careful clinicopathologic correlation.

Interpretation

- **Systemic lupus erythematosus (SLE)** – >95% of people with SLE have ANAs.

- **Healthy** – 5% of healthy people, particularly women, have ANAs.

- **Usefulness** – ANA test has high sensitivity, low specificity.

Specific Autoantibodies

- **Presence** – Many autoantibodies correlate with specific rheumatic diseases.

- **Outcomes** – In some instances, autoantibodies help predict disease prognosis or the occurrence of certain kinds of organ involvement. More often, however, these antibodies are markers for diagnosis and correlate only roughly (if at all) with disease activity or severity.

Complement

Values

- **Units** – U/ml.

- **Normal** – Depends on the reference ranges of the laboratory.

Interpretation

- **Decreased serum complement** – Often reflects active immune complex-mediated diseases (SLE).

- **Persistently low total hemolytic complement** – Suggests an inherited deficiency of a complement component.

- **Deficiencies of C1, C2, C3, or C4** – Increased susceptibility to SLE.

- **Acute-phase reactants** – Several complement components are acute-phase reactants. As such, their serum levels may rise during active inflammation.

Guidelines for Clinical Use of the Antinuclear Antibody Test

Conditions Associated with Positive IF-ANA Test Results[a]

Disease	Frequency of positive ANA result, %
Diseases for which an ANA test is very useful for diagnosis	
SLE	95–100
Systemic sclerosis (scleroderma)	60–80
Diseases for which an ANA test is somewhat useful for diagnosis	
Sjögren's syndrome	40–70
Idiopathic inflammatory myositis (dermatomyositis or polymyositis)	30–80
Diseases for which an ANA test is useful for monitoring or prognosis	
Juvenile chronic oligoarticular arthritis with uveitis	20–50
Raynaud's phenomenon	20–60
Conditions in which a positive ANA test result is an intrinsic part of the diagnostic criteria	
Drug-induced SLE	–100
Autoimmune hepatitis	–100
MCTD	–100

ANA, antinuclear antibody; IF, immunofluorescent; MCTD, mixed connective-tissue disease; SLE, systemic lupus erythematosus.

[a] Values are titers. Prevalence of positive ANA test result varies with titer. Female sex and increasing age tend to be more commonly associated with positive ANA.

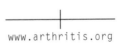

Disease	Frequency of positive ANA result, %
Diseases for which an ANA test is not useful in diagnosis	
Rheumatoid arthritis	30–50
Multiple sclerosis	25
Idiopathic thrombocytopenic purpura	10–30
Thyroid disease	30–50
Discoid lupus	5–25
Infectious diseases	Varies widely
Malignancies	Varies widely
Patients with silicone breast implants	15–25
Fibromyalgia	15–25
Relatives of patients with autoimmune diseases (SLE or scleroderma)	5–25
Normal persons	
≥1:40	20–30
≥1:80	10–12
≥1:160	5
≥1:320	3

Autoantibodies in Rheumatic Diseases

Type	Description
Anti-dsDNA	Antibodies to double-stranded DNA; greater specificity than those to single-stranded DNA
Anti-histone	Most assays do not differentiate the antibodies to the five major types of histones

Anti-ENA	Typical assays test for antibodies to two extractable nuclear antigens (ENAs):
	  Sm (Smith)
	  RNP (ribonucleoprotein)

Anti-SSA/Ro	Ribonucleoproteins
Anti-SSB/La	Ribonucleoproteins
Anti-centromere	Antibodies to the centromere/kinetochore region of the chromosome
Anti-Scl 70	Antibody to DNA topoisomerase I
Anti-Jo-1	Antibody to histidyl transfer RNA synthetase. The anti-Jo-1 antibody is the most common representative of a class of "myositis specific autoantibodies" known as anti-synthetase antibodies
Anti-PM-Scl	Antibodies to nucleolar granular component
Anti-Mi-2	Antibodies to a nucleolar antigen of unknown function

Clinical association

High specificity for SLE; occasionally appears in other illnesses and in normal people

SLE, drug-induced lupus, other autoimmune diseases

High specificity for SLE
MCTD, SLE

SLE (especially subacute cutaneous lupus), neonatal lupus, Sjögren's syndrome

Sjögren's syndrome, SLE, neonatal lupus

Limited scleroderma
(i.e., CREST syndrome)

Diffuse scleroderma

Poly/dermatomyositis; especially in patients with interstitial lung disease, Raynaud's phenomenon, cracked skin on hands ("mechanic's hands"), arthritis, and resistance to treatment

Polymyositis/scleroderma overlap syndrome

Dermatomyositis

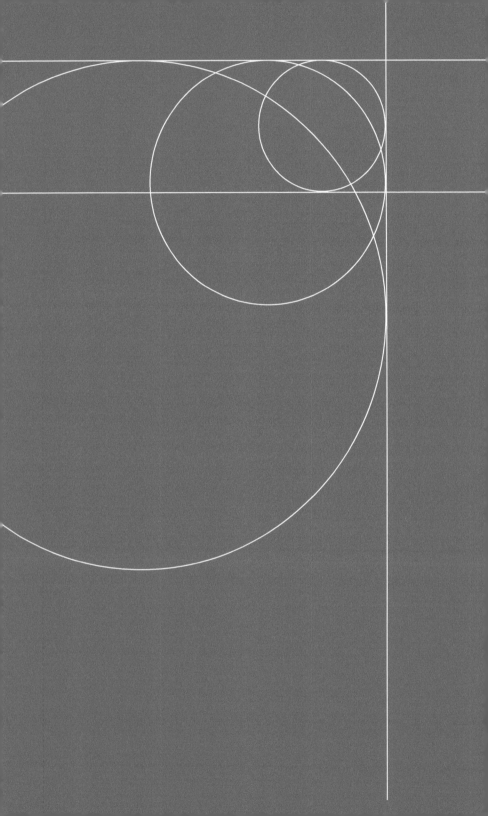

3 ARTHROCENTESIS AND SYNOVIAL FLUID ANALYSIS

Arthrocentesis and synovial fluid (SF) analysis yields valuable information that is important for the diagnosis of arthritis; arthrocentesis may help relieve signs and symptoms of arthritis, particularly if large joint effusions are present.

Indications

- **Infection** – Arthrocentesis must be performed immediately if there is any suspicion of infection. An inflammatory monarticular arthritis should be considered infectious until proven otherwise.

- **Crystal-induced disease** – Arthrocentesis and SF analysis are the only way to identify unequivocally.

- **Post-traumatic** – Analysis of joint fluid is the only way to distinguish post-traumatic hemarthrosis from post-traumatic arthritis with bland SF.

- **Inflammatory versus noninflammatory arthritides** – SF analysis enables the clinician to differentiate inflammatory and noninflammatory arthritides.

- **Therapeutic** – Arthrocentesis can be therapeutic, and can increase the efficacy of intra-articular glucocorticoids. Therapeutic arthrocentesis is indicated in any patient with a hemarthrosis.

Technique

- **Anesthesia** – Local anesthesia with 1% lidocaine without epinephrine significantly reduces discomfort associated with the procedure. A number 25 or 27 needle should be used to infiltrate the skin, subcutaneous tissue, and pericapsular tissue.

- **Needle choice** – After the periarticular tissues have been anesthetized, a 20- or 22-gauge needle can be used to aspirate small- to medium-sized joints. An 18- or 19-gauge needle should be used

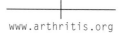

for aspirating large joints, if there is a suspicion of infection or intra-articular blood, or if there is a likelihood of viscous or loculated fluid.

- **Landmarks** – Typical landmarks often are obscured around a swollen joint. Therefore, after a thorough physical examination and before anesthetizing the skin, it is often helpful to mark the approach.

- **Position** – Unlike injection, aspiration is best done when a joint is in a position of maximum intra-articular pressure.

- **Radiographic assistance** – Although most joints can be aspirated without radiographic assistance, some joints, such as the hips, sacroiliac joints, or zygoapophyseal joints, require aspiration by an interventional radiologist under computed tomography guidance.

- **Collection** – SF should be collected in an EDTA or sodium heparin tube for cell counts, and a sterile tube for Gram stain and microbiology culture studies.

Classes of Synovial Fluid

Characteristic	Class I (noninflammatory)
Color	Clear/yellow
Clarity	Transparent
Viscosity	High
Mucin clot	Firm
WBC count	>2,000
Differential	<25% PMNs
Culture	Negative

PMNs, polymorphonuclear cells.

Anatomic Approach to Aspiration

Joint
Knee
Shoulder
Ankle
Subtalar
Wrist
First carpometacarpal
Metacarpophalangeal and interphalangeal
Metatarsophalangeal and interphalangeal
Elbow

Class II (inflammatory)	Class III (septic)	Class IV (hemorrhagic)
Yellow/white	Yellow/white	Red
Translucent/opaque	Opaque	Opaque
Variable	Low	Not applicable
Variable	Friable	Not applicable
2,000–100,000	>100,000	Not applicable
>50% PMNs	>95% PMNs	Not applicable
Negative	Positive	Variable

Position of the joint	Direction of the approach
Extended	Medial or lateral under the patella
Neutral adduction External rotation	Anterior: inferolateral to coracoid Posterior: under the acromion
Plantar flexion	Medial or lateral: anterior to the medial or lateral malleolus
Dorsiflexion to 90°	Inferior to tip of lateral malleolus
Midposition	Dorsal into radiocarpal joint
Thumb abducted and flexed	Proximal to base of the metacarpal
Finger slightly flexed	Just under extensor mechanism Dorsomedial or dorsolateral
Toes slightly flexed	Dorsomedial or dorsolateral
Flexed to 90°	Just under the lateral epicondyle

Diagnosis by Synovial Class

Class I	Class II
Osteoarthritis	Rheumatoid arthritis
Traumatic arthritis	Systemic lupus erythematosus
Osteonecrosis	Poly/dermatomyositis
Charcot's arthropathy	Scleroderma
	Systemic necrotizing vasculitides
	Polychondritis
	Gout
	CPPD deposition disease
	Hydroxyapatite deposition
	Juvenile rheumatoid arthritis
	Seronegative spondyloarthropathies
	Psoriatic arthritis
	Reactive arthritis
	Chronic inflammatory bowel disease
	Hypogammaglobulinemia
	Sarcoidosis
	Rheumatic fever
	Indolent/low virulence infections (viral, myobacterial, fungal, Whipple's disease, Lyme arthritis)

CPPD, calcium pyrophosphate dihydrate.

SF Analysis

- **Color** – Normal SF is colorless and clear. The yellow color characteristic of SF from people with arthritis is due to xanthochromia.

- **Opacity** – Generally, it is the number of white blood cells (WBCs) that determines the opacity of inflammatory SF. Synovial fluid from people with osteoarthritis is clear, whereas the SF in inflammatory arthropathies is translucent, and SF from a septic joint will be opaque.

- **Viscosity** – Normal joint fluid is viscous due to the presence of hyaluronic acid. Enzymes present in inflammatory arthropathies digest hyaluronic acid, resulting in a decrease in fluid viscosity.

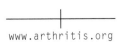

www.arthritis.org

Class III	Class IV
Bacterial arthritis	Trauma
	Pigmented villonodular synovitis
	Tuberculosis
	Tumor
	Coagulopathy
	Charcot's arthropathy

- **Blood** – The presence of blood in a joint usually is the result of acute trauma.

- **Crystals** – Although crystals can be identified in SF a few days old, optimal examinations for crystals are performed on wet preparations of SF soon after aspiration.

- **Classes** – There are four classes of SF, defined by differences in gross examination, total WBC count, WBC differential, the presence of absence of blood, and results of Gram stain and culture.

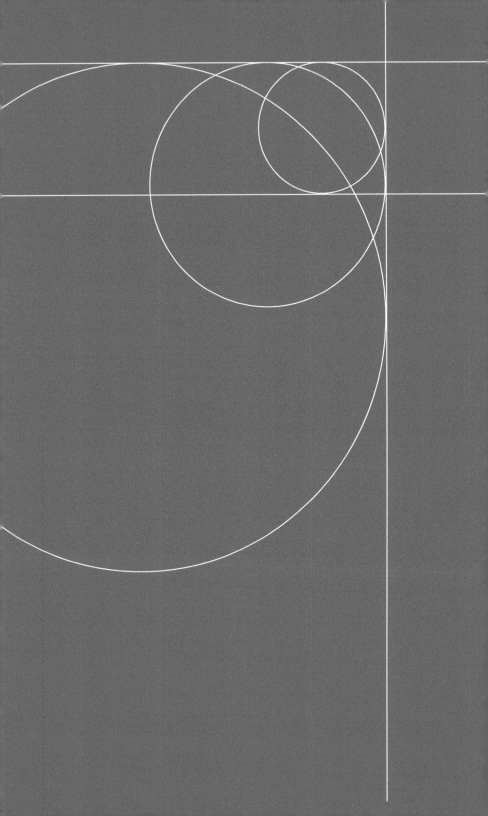

4 IMAGING TECHNIQUES

Imaging studies should not be obtained unless they have the potential to answer clinically significant questions. It is critically important for the clinician to work closely with the radiologist to decide exactly what information is needed to form an imaging study, and then to select the technique that will supply that information. Almost all imaging should begin with conventional radiography (plain X-rays).

Conventional Radiography

- **Starting point** – The conventional radiographic examination is the starting point for most imaging evaluations of arthritis.

- **Resolution** – Spatial resolution is very high, permitting good visualization of bony trabecular detail and tiny bone erosions. Contrast resolution is poor compared with computed tomography (CT) and magnetic resonance imaging (MRI).

- **Radiation** – Examination of peripheral structures delivers a low radiation dose. However, studies of central structures (spine and sacroiliac joints) expose patients to high radiation doses.

Computed Tomography

- **Availability** – CT is widely available, and many physicians are expert in its interpretation.

- **Resolution** – Spatial resolution is better than MRI, but inferior to that of conventional radiography.

- **Radiation** – The radiation dose from CT is relatively high, compared with a single plain radiograph of the same region, but is comparable when several conventional radiographic views of the same area are required.

- **Soft tissue** – CT demonstrates soft-tissue abnormalities far better than conventional radiography but not as well as MRI.

- **Disc disease** – CT is an excellent technique for evaluating degenerative disc disease of the spine and suspected disc herniations in older patients, in whom radiation dose is less critical than in young patients. High-quality MRI, if available, is preferred as the second study for investigating disc disease (following plain radiography), but CT is a good alternative and may be useful in circumstances where additional information about osteophytes is important.

- **Complex anatomy** – CT is useful for evaluating structures in areas of complex anatomy where overlying structures obscure the view on conventional radiographs.

Magnetic Resonance Imaging

- **Availability** – MRI is widely available, and expertise in its interpretation is growing rapidly.

- **Resolution** – Spatial resolution using the latest MRI equipment rivals that of CT, and contrast resolution in soft tissues is superior to that obtained by any other modality.

- **Radiation** – MRI is free of the hazards of ionizing radiation, a major advantage in examining central portions of the body.

- **Soft tissue** – MRI is able to image soft-tissue structures not visible on conventional radiographs. The menisci and cruciate ligaments of the knee, joint effusions, popliteal cysts, ganglion cysts, meniscal cysts, and bursitis are clearly imaged by MRI. The synovium can be imaged, especially using gadolinium.

- **Disc disease** – Although plain radiography is the initial method of evaluation in cases of suspected disc herniation, MRI also produces an excellent study of the spine and its contents.

- **Osteonecrosis (avascular necrosis)** – MRI is the study of choice for diagnosing early osteonecrosis.

Bone Densitometry

- **Use** – Bone densitometry is used primarily for evaluating osteoporosis.

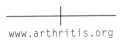

- **DEXA** – Dual emission X-ray absorptiometry.

  - **Radiation** – Very little radiation delivered to the patient. It is thus a good choice for studies that must be repeated.

  - **Structure studied** – Any part of the body can be studied, and standard values are available for lumbar spine and proximal femur, the most widely studied areas.

- **QCT** – Quantitative computed tomography.

  - **Radiation** – Radiation dose is fairly low, although not as low as that for DEXA.

  - **Structure studied** – One purported advantage of this technique is that it allows evaluation of cancellous bone in the middle of the vertebrae because it does not measure overlying cortical bone and posterior elements of the vertebrae.

Ultrasound

- **Availability** – Widely available.

- **Resolution** – Similar to CT and MRI, but is limited by the depth of tissue being studied.

- **Radiation** – No ionizing radiation.

- **Fluid collections** – Excellent for assessing joint effusions, popliteal cysts, and ganglion cysts. Can be used to guide aspiration of fluid in joints and elsewhere.

Scintigraphy

- **Availability** – At major medical centers.

- **Radiation** – Similar to CT scan of the abdomen.

- **99m technetium (^{99m}Tc) methylene disphosphonate** – Accumulates in areas of bone formation, calcium deposition, and high blood flow. Widely used for early detection of osteomyelitis.

- **^{99m}Tc sulfur colloid** – Localizes in the reticuloendothelial system (liver, spleen, and bone marrow).

- **67 gallium (^{67}Ga) citrate** – Accumulates in inflammatory and certain neoplastic processes.

- **111 indium (^{111}In)** – White blood cells labeled with ^{111}In localize inflammatory sites.

5 MONARTICULAR JOINT DISEASE

Pain or swelling of a single joint merits prompt evaluation to identify people in need of urgent and aggressive care.

- **Joint or soft-tissue disease** – Important to distinguish arthritis, which involves the articular space, from problems in periarticular areas, such as bursitis, tendinitis, or cellulitis.

- **Onset** – Sudden onset of monarthritis requires immediate evaluation and therapy.

- **Arthrocentesis** – Arthrocentesis and synovial fluid analysis should be performed in almost every person with monarthritis and a joint effusion, and it is *obligatory* if infection is suspected.

- **Causes** – The underlying causes of monarthritis are divided into two groups: inflammatory diseases and mechanical or infiltrative disorders.

- **Bacterial infection** – Generally associated with prominent inflammation. Symptoms tend to increase in severity until treated.

- **Viral monarthritis** – Often resolves spontaneously.

Some Inflammatory Causes of Monarthritis

Crystal-induced arthritis
Monosodium urate (gout)
Calcium pyrophosphate dihydrate
Apatite
Calcium oxalate
Liquid lipid microspherules
Infectious arthritis
Bacteria
Fungi
Lyme disease or disease due to other spirochetes
Mycobacteria
Virus (HIV, other)
Systemic diseases presenting with monarticular involvement
Psoriatic arthritis
Reactive arthritis
Rheumatoid arthritis
Systemic lupus erythematosus

- **Osteoarthritis** – Minimal or no inflammation; symptoms wax and wane with physical activity.

- **Inflammatory disease** – Morning stiffness lasting more than an hour suggests inflammatory disease.

- **Crystals** – Careful examination for crystals in synovial fluid can establish a diagnosis early.

Some Noninflammatory Causes of Monarthritis

Amyloidosis
Osteonecrosis
Benign tumor
  Osteochondroma
  Osteoid osteoma
  Pigmented villonodular synovitis
Fracture
Hemarthrosis
Internal derangement
Malignancy
Osteoarthritis

6 POLYARTICULAR JOINT DISEASE

A thorough history and physical examination are the most important diagnostic tools in the evaluation of polyarticular joint complaints.

- **Patterns** – Determine the pattern and evolution of joint involvement and the pattern of pain.

- **Joint examination** – Note the presence of joint effusions, tenderness, range of motion, and soft-tissue swelling.

- **Spine and muscles** – Examine the spine and muscles as well as the joints.

- **Skin** – Give particular attention to examining the skin for rashes, subcutaneous nodules, and other lesions associated with rheumatic diseases.

- **Laboratory tests** – Laboratory studies should be directed by suspected diagnoses elicited by history and physical examination. These include standard hematologic and biochemical tests; acute-phase reactants (ESR or CRP); and autoantibody tests. Autoantibodies may be associated with a single condition or limited group of illnesses.

- **Synovial fluid** – Examine synovial fluid if it is readily obtainable, and in particular if the diagnosis is uncertain after history, physical examination, and results of standard laboratory tests.

- **Imaging** – Rarely indicated or helpful in acute polyarthritis, but important in chronic polyarthritis (greater than eight weeks). Plain radiographs useful to identify abnormalities of bone and cartilage.

- **Narrow the choices** – Outline the differential diagnosis and estimate the likelihood that a test or study will distinguish between the leading diagnoses or alter the treatment plan.

- **Articular causes** – There are two main categories of polyarticular joint disease: inflammatory and noninflammatory.

- **Nonarticular causes** – Consider nonarticular causes if the joints appear normal in patients with widespread pain (e.g., fibromyalgia, polymyalgia rheumatica, bone disease, neuropathy).

Classification of Inflammatory Polyarticular Joint Disease

Crystal-induced arthritis	Rheumatoid arthritis
Infectious arthritis	Inflammatory osteoarthritis
Bacterial	Systemic rheumatic illnesses
Gonococcal and meningococcal	Systemic lupus erythematosus
Lyme disease	Systemic vasculitis
Bacterial endocarditis	Polymyositis/dermatomyositis
Viral	Still's disease
Other infections	Behçet's syndrome
Postinfectious or reactive arthritis	Relapsing polychondritis
Enteric infection	Other systemic illnesses
Urogenital infection	Sarcoidosis
Rheumatic fever	Palindromic rheumatism
Other seronegative spondyloarthropathies	Familial Mediterranean fever
Ankylosing spondylitis	Malignancy
Psoriatic arthritis	Hyperlipoproteinemias
Inflammatory bowel disease	Whipple's disease

Classification of Noninflammatory Polyarticular Joint Disease

Osteoarthritis	Hematologic
Metabolic/endocrine	Amyloidosis
Hemochromatosis	Leukemia
Acromegaly	Hemophilia
Ochronosis	Sickle cell disease
	Hypertrophic pulmonary osteoarthropathy

7 REGIONAL RHEUMATIC PAIN SYNDROMES

Regional rheumatic pain syndromes present challenges to the clinician because of their prevalence, complexity, and lack of diagnostic laboratory tests. A precise history starts any work-up. In addition, a complete musculoskeletal examination should be performed, emphasizing careful palpation, passive range of motion (ROM), active ROM, and sometimes, active ROM with resistance. Treating regional pain focuses on patient education, pain management, and physical therapy.

Guidelines for Management of Regional Rheumatic Pain Syndromes

1. Exclude systemic disease and infection by appropriate methods. Diagnostic aspiration is mandatory in suspected septic bursitis. Gram stain and culture of bursal fluid provide prompt diagnosis of a septic bursitis.

2. Teach the patient to recognize and avoid aggravating factors that cause recurrences.

3. Instruct the patient in self-help therapy, including the daily performance of mobilizing exercises.

4. Provide an explanation of the cause of pain, thus alleviating concern for a crippling disease. When the regional rheumatic pain syndrome overlies another rheumatic problem, the clinician must explain the contribution each disorder plays in the symptom complex and then help the patient deal with each one.

5. Provide relief from pain with safe analgesics, counterirritants (heat, ice, vapocoolant sprays), and if appropriate, intralesional injection of a local anesthetic, or anesthetic with depository glucocorticoid agent.

6. Provide the patient with an idea of the duration of therapy necessary to restore order to the musculoskeletal system.

7. Symptomatic relief often corroborates the diagnosis.

Disorders of the Lower Back

- **Various causes** – The symptom of axial skeleton pain is associated with a wide variety of mechanical and medical disorders.

- **Mechanical causes** – Mechanical disorders are the most common causes of low back pain.

- **Rheumatic causes** – Rheumatic causes of low back pain include OA, ankylosing spondylitis, and spondyloarthropathies.

- **Sciatica** – Intervertebral disc herniation causes nerve impingement and inflammation that result in radicular pain (sciatica).

- **Treatment** – Acute low back pain can be treated using the Agency for Health Care Policy and Research Guidelines.

Disorders Affecting the Low Back and/or Neck

Mechanical
Muscle strain
Herniated intervertebral disc
Osteoarthritis
Spinal stenosis
Spinal stenosis with myelopathy*
Spondylolysis/spondylolisthesis+
Adult scoliosis+
Whiplash*

Rheumatologic
Ankylosing spondylitis
Reiter's syndrome
Psoriatic arthritis
Enteropathic arthritis
Rheumatoid arthritis*
Diffuse idiopathic skeletal hyperostosis
Vertebral osteochondritis+
Polymyalgia rheumatica
Fibromyalgia
Behçet's syndrome+
Whipple's disease+
Hidradenitis suppurativa+
Osteitis condensans ilii+

Endocrinologic/metabolic
Osteoporosis+
Osteomalacia+
Parathyroid disease+
Microcrystalline disease
Ochronosis+
Fluorosis+
Heritable genetic disorders

* Neck predominant.
+ Low back predominant.

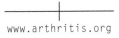

Neurologic/psychiatric
Neuropathic arthropathy[+]
Neuropathies
   Tumors
   Vasculitis
   Compression
Psychogenic rheumatism
Depression
Malingering

Miscellaneous
Paget's disease
Vertebral sarcoidosis
Subacute bacterial endocarditis[+]
Retroperitoneal fibrosis[+]

Infectious
Vertebral osteomyelitis
Meningitis[+]
Discitis
Pyogenic sacroiliitis[+]
Herpes zoster
Lyme disease

Neoplastic/infiltrative
Benign tumors
   Osteoid osteoma[+]
   Osteoblastoma
   Osteochondroma
   Giant cell tumor
   Aneurysmal bone cyst
   Hemangioma
   Eosinophilic granuloma
   Gaucher's disease[+]
   Sacroiliac lipoma[+]

Malignant tumors
   Skeletal metastases
   Multiple myeloma
   Chondrosarcoma
   Chordoma
   Lymphoma[+]
Intraspinal lesions
   Metastases
   Meningioma
   Vascular malformations
   Gliomas
   Syringomyelia[+]

Hematologic
Hemoglobinopathies[+]
Myelofibrosis[+]
Mastocytosis[+]

Referred pain
Vascular
   Abdominal aorta[+]
   Cartoid*
   Thoracic aorta*
Gastrointestinal
   Pancreas
   Gallbladder
   Intestine
   Esophagus*

Genitourinary[+]
Kidney
Ureter
Bladder
Uterus
Ovary
Prostrate

Modified with permission from Borenstein DG, Wiesel SW, Boden SD. Low Back Pain: Medical Diagnosis and Comprehensive Management, 2nd edition. Philadelphia, PA: W.B. Saunders, 1995, copyright © 1995. And from Borenstein DG, Wiesel SW, Boden SD. Neck Pain: Medical Diagnosis and Comprehensive Management. Philadelphia, PA: W.B. Saunders, 1996, copyright © 1996.

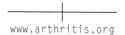

Radicular Symptoms and Signs

Pain distribution	
Lumbar	
4	Anterior thigh to medial leg
5	Lateral leg to dorsum of foot
S1	Lateral foot
Cervical	
5	Neck to outer shoulder, arm
6	Outer arm to thumb, index fingers
7	Outer arm to middle fingers
8	Inner arm to ring, little fingers

AHCPR Guidelines for Acute Low Back Pain Treatment

Patient education

Natural history of rapid recovery and recurrence

Safe and effective methods of symptom control

Activity modifications

Limit recurrences

Special investigations required with systemic disorders suspected

Risks of common diagnostic tests

Treatment recommendations for persistent symptoms

Medications

Acetaminophen

NSAIDs: decision based on comorbidities, toxicities, cost, patient preferences

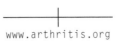

www.arthritis.org

Sensory loss	Motor loss	Reflex loss
Medial leg to medial malleolus	Anterior tibialis	Patellar
Lateral leg to dorsum of foot	Extensor hallucis longus	(Posterior tibial)
Lateral foot, sole	Peroneus longus and brevis	Achilles
Shoulder	Deltoid	Biceps, supinator
Thumb, index fingers	Biceps, wrist extensors	Biceps, supinator
Index, middle fingers	Triceps	Triceps
Ring, little fingers	Hand muscles	None

Physical treatments

Spinal manipulation in the first month in the absence of radiculopathy (efficacy short term)

Activity modification

Bed rest no more than four days

Gradual return to normal activities

Low-stress aerobic exercise

Mechanical Disorders of the Low Back

Disorder	Signs/symptoms
Back strain	Acute-onset back pain usually preceded by trauma; pain radiates up the ipsilateral paraspinous muscles, across the lumbar area, and sometimes caudally to the buttocks
Herniated nucleus pulposus	Acute-onset chronic lumbar pain that increases when sitting and bending, decreases when standing
Osteoarthritis	Insidious-onset chronic lumbar pain that increases at the end of the day and radiates across the low back
Spinal stenosis	Insidious-onset leg pain, pattern of radiation depends on location of nerve compression
Spondylolisthesis	Insidious-onset low back pain; pain increases with standing, relieved with rest
Adult scoliosis	Increasing back pain relieved with bed rest

Disorders of the Neck

Disorder	Signs/symptoms
Neck strain	Acute-onset pain in the middle or lower part of the posterior aspect of the neck; pain may radiate toward head and/or shoulder
Herniated nucleus pulposus	Radicular pain that radiates from the shoulder to the forearm to the hand; neck pain minimal or absent
Osteoarthritis	Insidious-onset diffuse neck pain that may radiate to shoulders, suboccipital areas, interscapular muscles, or anterior chest
Myelopathy	Sensory abnormalities in the hands associated with weakness and uncoordination
Whiplash	Stiffness and pain with motion after auto accident; headache common

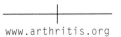

Diagnostic clues	Notes
Pain increases when standing and bending, decreases when sitting; straight leg raising does not induce pain; limited ROM in lumbar area	Imaging not necessary
Straight leg raising, sitting, bending, and Valsalva's maneuver elicit radicular pain; pain decreases when standing	MRI is best technique to locate disc herniation and nerve impingement
Pain worsens with extension of the spine; straight leg raising does not induce pain	
Pain is relieved when patient sits or flexes forward; straight leg raising induces pain	MRI can document the location of the neural compression
Increased lordosis with a "stepoff"; straight leg raising does not induce pain	Plain radiographs can document the lesion; MRI can detect nerve entrapment and impingement
Neurologic exam reveals nerve compression in severe cases	Plain radiographs allow measurement of degree of scoliosis curvature

Diagnostic clues	Notes
Local tenderness in the paracervical muscles. Decreased ROM and loss of cervical lordosis	Imaging not necessary
Lateral flexion and extension cause radicular pain; neurologic exam may reveal sensory deficit, reflex asymmetry, or motor weakness	MRI identifies location of disc herniation and nerve impingement
Exam reveals little other than midline tenderness	Plain radiographs adequate
Decreased dermatomal sensation and loss of proprioception	Plain radiographs reveal advanced degenerative disease; MRI will detect extent of spinal compression; progressive myelopathy requires surgery
Decreased neck ROM; persistent paracervical muscle contraction	Imaging not necessary

Disorders of the Shoulder Region

Disorder	Signs/symptoms
Rotator cuff tendinitis	Shoulder pain, usually over the lateral deltoid
Rotator cuff tear	Shoulder pain, weakness and/or pain on abduction, loss of motion, night pain, tenderness on palpation
Bicipital tendinitis	Pain in the anterior region of the shoulder
Adhesive capsulitis	Generalized shoulder pain; severe loss of active and passive motion in all planes
Thoracic outlet syndrome	Pain, paresthesia, and numbness radiating from the neck and shoulder down to the arm and hand; activity worsens symptoms

Disorders of the Elbow Region

Disorder	Signs/symptoms
Olecranon bursitis	Bursa swollen and tender on pressure; pain minimal and ROM preserved
Lateral epicondylitis (tennis elbow)	Localized tenderness over or slightly anterior to the lateral epicondyle
Medial epicondylitis (golfer's elbow)	Localized pain and tenderness over the medial epicondyle

Diagnostic clues	Notes
Pain with active abduction (60°–120°) and internal rotation; positive impingement sign	Injection of depot glucocorticoid into the subacromial bursa
Positive drop-arm sign (large tears); abnormal arthrogram, diagnostic ultrasound, and MRI can all be used to identify cuff tears	Surgical repair for large tears in young patients
Pain reproduced by supination of forearm against resistance	Subluxation of rupture of tendon possible
Arthrography shows decreased shoulder joint capsule volume and loss of normal axillary pouch	Inflammatory arthritis and diabetes possible causes
Weakened radial pulse with neck extension and rotations	Weakness and atrophy of intrinsic muscles are late findings; vascular symptoms are discoloration, temperature change, pain on use, and Raynaud's phenomenon

Diagnostic clues	Notes
Aspiration yields clear or bloody fluid with a low viscosity	Inflammatory or septic bursitis possible; aspirate and culture
Resisted wrist extension aggravates the pain	
Resisted wrist flexion exacerbates the pain	

Disorders of the Wrist and Hand

Disorder	Signs/symptoms
Ganglion	Swelling over the dorsum of the wrist
DeQuervain's tenosynovitis	Pain, tenderness, and occasionally swelling over the radial styloid
Tenosynovitis of the wrist	Localized pain and tenderness, sometimes swelling
Radial nerve palsy	Anesthesia in the web space and hyperesthesia from the dorsal aspect of the forearm to the thumb, index, and middle fingers
Carpal tunnel syndrome	Burning pain or tingling in the hand, usually at night, relieved by vigorous shaking of the hand; numbness
Dupuytren's contracture	Initially, mildly tender fibrous nodule in the volar fascia of the palm; later, thick cord-like superficial fibrous tissue in the palm

Disorders of the Hip Region

Disorder	Signs/symptoms
Trochanteric bursitis	Aching over the trochanteric area and lateral thigh
Iliopsoas (iliopectineal) bursitis	Groin and anterior thigh pain, which worsens on passive hyperextension of the hip and sometimes on flexion
Ischial (ischiogluteal) bursitis	Exquisite pain when sitting or lying down; may radiate down back of thigh
Piriformis syndrome	Pain over the buttocks, often radiating down the back of the leg
Meralgia paresthetica	Intermittent burning pain, associated with hypesthesia and sometimes with numbness of the anterolateral thigh

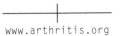

Diagnostic clues	Notes
	If needed, treat with aspiration with or without glucocorticoid injection
Inflammation and narrowing of the tendon sheath around the abductor pollicis longus and extensor pollicis brevis; pain with folding thumb in palm, and ulnar deviation of wrist (Finkelstein test)	Finkelstein test also positive in OA of the first carpometacarpal joint
Pain on resisted movement	May be misinterpreted as arthritis
Wrist-drop with flexion of the MCP joints and adduction of the thumb	Most common in spiral groove syndrome (bridegroom palsy)
Positive Tinel's sign or Phalen's sign; prolonged distal latency during electrodiagnostic studies	Surgical decompression may be necessary if conservative treatment fails
Dimpling or puckering of the skin over the fascia helps identify this disorder	

Diagnostic clues	Notes
Point tenderness on palpation of the trochanteric area; additional tender points may be noted throughout lateral thigh muscle	Walking and lying on involved side may intensify pain
Tenderness palpable over involved bursa; diagnosis confirmed by plain radiography and injection of contrast medium into bursa, or by CT or MRI	Patient may hold hip in flexion and external rotation to eliminate pain
Point tenderness over the ischial tuberosity	Caused by trauma or prolonged sitting on hard surface
Tenderness of the piriformis muscle on rectal or vaginal exam; pain evident on internal rotation of the hips against resistance	
Touch and pinprick sensation over the anterolateral thigh may be decreased; pain elicited by pressing on the inguinal ligament just medial to the anterior superior iliac spine	

Disorders of the Knee Region

Disorder	Signs/symptoms
Popliteal cysts (Baker's cyst)	Diffuse swelling and tenderness of popliteal space
Anserine bursitis	Pain and knee tenderness over the medial aspect of the knee, about 5 cm below the joint margin
Prepatellar bursitis	Swelling superficial to the kneecap
Patellar tendinitis (jumper's knee)	Pain and tenderness over the patellar tendon
Rupture of quadriceps tendon and infrapatellar tendon	Sudden sharp pain and inability to extend leg
Peroneal nerve palsy	Painless foot drop with a steppage gait
Patellofemoral pain syndrome	Pain and crepitus in the patellar region; stiffness after prolonged sitting; alleviated by activity

Disorders of the Anterior Chest Wall

Disorder	Signs/symptoms
Tietze's syndrome	Pain may radiate to the shoulder, aggravated by coughing, sneezing, inspiration
Costochondritis	Pain and tenderness of the chest wall

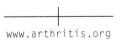

Diagnostic clues	Notes
Seen best with patient standing and examined from behind; ultrasound, MRI, or arthrogram may be useful in diagnosis	Possibility of dissection or rupture causing swelling or erythema in calf. This can mimic a deep venous thrombosis
Exquisite tenderness elicited over the bursa and relieved with local lidocaine injection	Often seen in people with obese legs and OA of the knees
Pain elicited when pressure is applied directly over bursa	Consider septic prepatellar bursitis when erythema, heat, and increased tenderness and pain are present
	Glucocorticoid injections contraindicated
Radiographs may show a high-riding patella	Surgical repair necessary
Pain sensation decreased slightly along the lower lateral aspect of the leg and dorsum of foot; nerve conduction studies show decreases in conduction velocities	
Pain elicited when patella is compressed against the femoral condyle or when patella is displaced laterally	

Diagnostic clues	Notes
Swelling in the second or third costal cartilage; tenderness on palpation	
Lack of swelling; tenderness present over more than one costochondral junction; palpation duplicates described pain	

Disorders of the Ankle and Foot Region

Disorder	Signs/symptoms
Achilles tendinitis	Pain, swelling, and tenderness over the Achilles tendon
Retrocalcaneal bursitis	Pain at back of heel, tenderness anterior to the Achilles tendon, pain on dorsiflexion
Plantar fasciitis	Pain in the plantar area of the heel; pain worse in morning upon rising
Achilles tendon rupture	Sudden or subacute onset of pain during forced dorsiflexion; audible snap may be heard; difficulty walking and standing on toes
Tarsal tunnel syndrome	Numbness, burning pain, and paresthesias of the toes and sole extend proximally to the area over the medial malleolus; relief with leg, foot, and ankle movements
Hallux valgus	Bunion on the head of the first MTP joint causing pain, tenderness, and swelling
Bunionette	Prominence of the fifth metatarsal head
Hammertoe	Tip of toe points downward; calluses at tip of toe and over dorsum of IP joint
Morton's neuroma	Paresthesia and a burning, aching pain in the fourth toes; symptoms made worse by walking on hard surfaces or wearing tight shoes
Metatarsalgia	Pain on standing, calluses over the metatarsal heads
Pes planus	Fatigue of the foot muscle and aching, intolerance to prolonged walking or standing
Pes cavus	Claw-like appearance of the toes; calluses over the dorsum of the toes; foot fatigue, pain, and tenderness of the metatarsal heads

Diagnostic clues	Notes
Crepitus on motion and pain on dorsiflexion	Usually caused by trauma or overactivity; can be caused by inflammatory rheumatic conditions
Local swelling with bulging on the medial and lateral aspect of the tendon	May be secondary to RA, spondylitis, reactive arthritis, gout, or trauma
Palpation reveals tenderness anteromedially on the medial calcaneal tubercle at the origin of the plantar fascia	
Weakness and absence of plantar flexion; MRI helpful in diagnosis	Orthopaedic consultation required
Loss of pinprick and two-point discrimination	
Deviation of the large toe lateral to the midline and deviation of the first metatarsal medially	
Fifth metatarsal has a lateral deviation	
PIP joint is flexed	
Tenderness elicited by palpation between third and fourth metatarsal heads	Surgical excision may be needed if conservative therapy ineffective
Tenderness on palpation of the metatarsal heads	
Flattening of the transverse arch and weakness of the intrinsic muscles, maldistribution of weight on forefoot	Flatfoot
Unusually high medial arch, shortening of the extensor ligaments; dorsiflexion of the PIP joints and plantar flexion of the DIP joints	Clawfoot

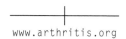

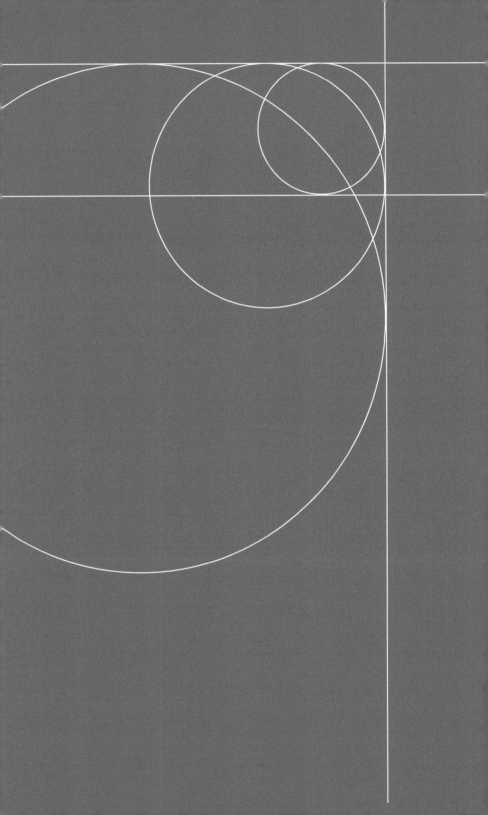

8 FIBROMYALGIA AND DIFFUSE PAIN SYNDROMES

Clinical Features

- **Pain** – The pain frequently waxes and wanes, may be migratory, and often is accompanied by dysesthias or paresthesias following a nondermatomal distribution.

- **Regional musculoskeletal pain** – Regional pain typically involves the axial skeleton or areas of tender points, and originally may be diagnosed as a local problem.

- **Regional nonmusculoskeletal pain** – Other associated symptoms include a higher-than-expected prevalence of tension and migraine headaches, temporomandibular joint syndrome, non-cardiac chest pain, irritable bowel syndrome, several entities characterized by chronic pelvic pain, and plantar or heel pain.

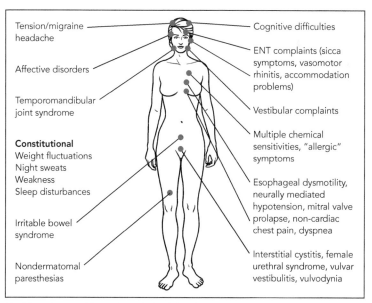

Nondefining features of fibromyalgia and related disorders.

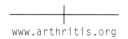

- **Physical examination** – Physical exam generally is unremarkable, except for tender points in fibromyalgia

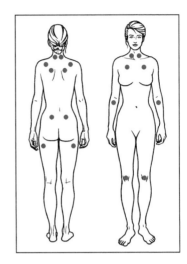

The location of the nine paired tender points that comprise the 1990 American College of Rheumatology criteria for fibromyalgia.

Diagnosis

- **Differential diagnosis** – many different conditions can simulate fibromyalgia and other chronic pain syndromes.

Conditions that Stimulate Fibromyalgia, or Occur Concurrently with Fibromyalgia

Common
Hypothyroidism Medications (especially lipid-lowering drugs, antiviral agents) Polymyalgia rheumatica Hepatitis C Sleep apnea Parvovirus infection Cervical stenosis/Chiari malformation
Less common
Autoimmune disorders (e.g., SLE, RA, especially early in course of disease) Endocrine disorders e.g., Addison's disease, Cushing's syndrome, hyperparathyroidism) Lyme disease Eosinophilia-myalgia syndrome Glucocorticoid use Malignancy

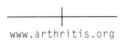

- **Fibromyalgia criteria** – to fulfill the 1990 ACR criteria for fibromyalgia, an individual must have a history of chronic widespread pain involving all four quadrants of the body (and the axial skeleton) and the presence of 11 to 18 "tender points" on physical examination. At least half of the individuals who have the clinical diagnosis of fibromyalgia will not fulfill the ACR definition.

Criteria for the Classification of Fibromyalgia

1. History of widespread pain
Definition. Pain is considered widespread when all of the following are present: pain in the left side of the body, pain in the right side of the body, pain above the waist, and pain below the waist. In addition, axial skeletal pain (cervical spine or anterior chest or thoracic spine or low back) must be present. In this definition, shoulder and buttock pain is considered as pain for each involved side. "Low back" pain is considered lower segment pain.
2. Pain in 11 of 18 tender point sites on digital palpation
Definition. Pain, on digital palpation, must be present in at least 11 of the following 18 tender point sites: *Occiput:* bilateral, at the suboccipital muscle insertions   *Low cervical:* bilateral, at the anterior aspects of the intertransverse spaces at C5–C7   *Trapezius:* bilateral, at the midpoint of the upper border   *Supraspinatus:* bilateral, at origins, above the scapula spine near the medial border   *Second rib:* bilateral, at the second costochondral junctions, just lateral to the junctions on upper surfaces   *Lateral epicondyle:* bilateral, 2 cm distal to the epicondyles   *Gluteal:* bilateral, in upper outer quadrants of buttocks in anterior fold of muscle   *Greater trochanter:* bilateral, posterior to the trochanteric prominence   *Knee:* bilateral, at the medial fat pad proximal to the joint line

For classification purposes, patients will be said to have fibromyalgia if both criteria are satisfied. Widespread pain must have been present at least 3 months. The presence of a second clinical disorder does not exclude the diagnosis of fibromyalgia. Digital palpation should be performed with an approximate force of 4 kg. For a tender point to be considered "positive," the subject must state that the palpation was painful. "Tender" is not to be considered "painful."

Adapted from Wolfe F, Smythe HA, Yunus MB, et al. The American College of Rheumatology 1990 criteria for the classification of fibromyalgia. Report of the multicenter criteria committee. Arthritis Rheum 1990; 33: 160–172. Copyright © 1990 American College of Rheumatology. Reproduced with permission of John Wiley & Sons, Inc.

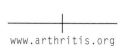

- **Exclude autoimmune disorders** – Symptoms that may be seen in both fibromyalgia and autoimmune disorders include not only arthralgias, myalgias, and fatigue, but also morning stiffness and subjective swelling of the hands and feet. In addition, a Raynaud's-like syndrome (characterized by the entire hand turning pale or red, instead of just the digits), malar flushing (in contrast to a fixed malar rash), and livedo reticularis are common in fibromyalgia and can mislead the practitioner to suspect an autoimmune disorder.

Treatment

- **Spend time** – Schedule a prolonged visit or series of visits when this diagnosis is considered.

- **Explore the symptoms** – Discuss the most bothersome, the impact these symptoms are having on various aspects of life, perception about what is causing these symptoms, and the stressors that may be exacerbating the problem.

- **Educate** – Provide information about the nature of this disorder.

- **Begin treatment program** – Combine symptom-based pharmacologic therapy with extensive use of nonpharmacologic therapies.

- **Nonpharmacologic therapy** – Cognitive-behavioral therapy and aerobic exercise have been most effective.

- **Tricyclic drugs** – Among the many drugs that have been used to treat fibromyalgia, tricyclic drugs are the most noteworthy. To increase the tolerance of cyclobenzaprine and amitriptyline, these compounds should be administered several hours before bedtime, begun at low doses (10 mg or less), and increased slowly (10 mg every one to two weeks) until the patient reaches the maximally beneficial dose (up to 40 mg of cyclobenzaprine, or 70–80 mg of amitriptyline).

- **Complementary therapies** – These therapies include trigger-point injections, myofascial release therapy (or other "hands-on" techniques), acupuncture, and chiropractic manipulation, each of which has some data supporting efficacy.

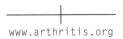

9 RHEUMATOID ARTHRITIS

Clinical Features

Articular Manifestations

- **Two categories** – Articular manifestations can be divided into two categories: reversible symptoms and signs related to inflammatory synovitis, and irreversible damage caused by structural changes in the synovium, bone, cartilage, and other joint structures.

- **Morning stiffness** – An almost universal feature of synovial inflammation. Morning stiffness in untreated rheumatoid arthritis (RA) usually lasts more than 2 hours.

- **Signs of synovitis** – Warm, swollen, grossly inflamed joints usually are detected only in the most active phases of inflammatory synovitis. In chronic disease, granulation tissue and fibrosis develop, and the degree of inflammation is reduced.

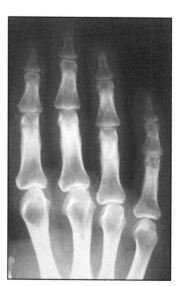

- **Structural damage** – Cartilage loss and erosion of periarticular bone are the characteristic features of structural damage. Clinical features related to structural damage are marked by joint deformity and loss of joint function.

In rheumatoid arthritis, periarticular osteopenia is an early radiological feature.

Joints Affected by RA

Cervical spine	Neck stiffness and general loss of motion
Shoulders	Shoulder effusions are difficult to detect on physical examination except in cases of advanced shoulder dysfunction. Warmth may be felt over acutely inflamed joints, but often the only objective findings are pain with joint movements and reduction in the normal range of motion
Elbow	Synovitis is indicated by fullness and thickening of the radiohumeral joint on palpation
Hand and wrist	Wrists are affected in virtually all people with RA. MCP and PIP joints are often involved; the DIPs usually are spared
Hip	Hip involvement is common in RA, but early manifestations may be difficult to detect
Knee	Effusions and synovial thickening of the knee usually are identified easily. If a knee is not cooler than its ipsilateral shin, a joint effusion is probably present
Foot and ankle	RA characteristically affects the MTP, talonavicular, and ankle joints

MCP, metacarpophalangeal; PIP, proximal interphalangeal; DIP, distal interphalangeal; MTP, metatarsophalangeal.

Extra-Articular Manifestations

- **Constitutional symptoms** – RA is a systemic disease. Most patients experience general malaise or fatigue. Fever and weight loss may occur.

- **Organs** – A host of other organs can be involved in RA. Extra-articular disease is more likely among seropositive patients, i.e. those whose serum contains either rheumatoid factor (RF) or antibodies directed against cyclic citrullinated peptides (anti-CCP antibodies).

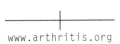

Organ Systems Affected by RA

Skin	Rheumatoid nodules among 50% of RA patients, particularly those who are seropositive. The skin may also demonstrate features of rheumatoid vasculitis, especially cutaneous nodules and ulcers
Eyes	Keratoconjunctivitis sicca, episcleritis, scleritis, keratitis, and corneal melt occur
Lungs	Interstitial lung disease is common, but may be asymptomatic
Heart	Pericardial effusion is present among almost 50% of patients, but clinical symptoms are rare
Nervous system	Effects follow cervical spine instability, peripheral nerve entrapment, and vasculitis resulting in mononeuritis multiplex
Blood	Normochromic, normocytic anemia consistent with an anemia of chronic disease. This process is characterized by a low concentration of serum iron, a low serum iron-binding capacity, and a normal or increased serum ferritin concentration

Laboratory Features

- **Rheumatoid factor** – RF is found in the serum of approximately 85% of people with RA. RF is a marker for patients with more aggressive disease, who are at greater risk for joint destruction and extra-articular disease compared with patients who are RF-negative.

- **Anti-CCP antibodies** – Anti-CCP antibodies are slightly more sensitive than RF and substantially more specific for RA. They also serve as a marker for patients predisposed to aggressive disease. Neither RF nor anti-CCP antibodies, however, correlate well with disease activity.

- **Acute-phase reactants** – The erythrocyte sedimentation rate (ESR) and C-reactive protein (CRP) correlate with the degree of synovial inflammation. They are useful for following the course of inflammatory activity in an individual patient.

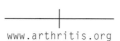

www.arthritis.org

- **Other laboratory tests** – Abnormalities include hypergamma-globulinemia, thrombocytosis, anemia, and neutropenia. These occur more often among patients with severe disease, high RF titer, rheumatoid nodules and extra-articular manifestations.

Diagnosis

- **Exclusions** – Diagnosis during the early weeks of inflammatory arthritis is one of exclusion of other inflammatory polyarticular joint diseases.

Inflammatory Polyarticular Joint Diseases

Crystal-induced arthritis	Rheumatoid arthritis
Infectious arthritis	Inflammatory osteoarthritis
Bacterial	Systemic rheumatic illnesses
Gonococcal and meningococcal	Systemic lupus erythematosus
Lyme disease	Systemic vasculitis
Bacterial endocarditis	Systemic sclerosis
Viral (particularly parvovirus B19)	Polymyositis/dermatomyositis
Other infections	Still's disease
Postinfectious or reactive arthritis	Behçet's disease
Enteric infection	Other systemic illnesses
Urogenital infection	Sarcoidosis
Rheumatic fever	Palindromic rheumatism
Other seronegative spondyloarthropathies	Familial Mediterranean fever
Ankylosing spondylitis	Malignancy
Psoriatic arthritis	Hyperlipoproteinemias
Inflammatory bowel disease	Whipple's disease

- **Characteristic features** – Symmetric synovitis of small joints of the hands and feet with typical serologic findings strongly suggest RA. The larger joints of the wrists, elbows, shoulders, neck, hips, knees, and ankles can also be affected. Symmetrical disease is the rule.

- **Erosions** – Radiographic evidence of erosions becomes apparent only after several months or more than a year.

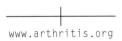

American College of Rheumatology Criteria for the Classification of Rheumatoid Arthritis

Criterion	Definition
1. Morning stiffness	Morning stiffness in and around the joints, lasting at least 1 hour before maximal improvement
2. Arthritis of three or more joint areas	At least three joint areas simultaneously have had soft-tissue swelling or fluid (not bony overgrowth alone) observed by a physician. The 14 possible areas are right or left PIP, MCP, wrist, elbow, knee, ankle, and MTP joints
3. Arthritis of hand joints	At least one area swollen (as defined above) in a wrist, MCP, or PIP joint
4. Symmetric arthritis	Simultaneous involvement of the same joint areas (as defined in 2) on both sides of the body (bilateral involvement of PIPs, MCPs, or MTPs is acceptable. Absolute symmetry not required)
5. Rheumatoid nodules	Subcutaneous nodules over bony prominences or extensor surfaces, or in juxta-articular regions, observed by a physician. Rheumatoid nodules can also occur in visceral organs, e.g. the lung
6. Serum rheumatoid factor	Demonstration of abnormal amounts of rheumatoid factor by any method for which the result has been positive in <5% of normal control subjects
7. Radiographic changes	Radiographic changes typical of rheumatoid arthritis on posteroanterior hand and wrist, which must include erosions or unequivocal bony decalcification localized in or most marked adjacent to the involved joints (osteoarthritis changes alone do not qualify)

For classification purposes, a patient shall be said to have rheumatoid arthritis if he/she has satisfied at least four of these seven criteria. Criteria 1 through 4 must have been present for at least 6 weeks. Patients with two clinical diagnoses are not excluded. Designation as classic, definite, or probable rheumatoid arthritis is not to be made.

Reprinted from Arnett FC, Edworthy SM, Bloch DA, et al. The American Rheumatism Association 1987 revised criteria for the classification of Rheumatology. Arthritis Rheum 1988; 31: 315–324. Copyright © 1988 American College of Rheumatology. Reproduced with permission of John Wiley & Sons, Inc.

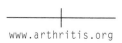

www.arthritis.org

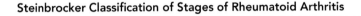

Steinbrocker Classification of Stages of Rheumatoid Arthritis

Stage I, Early
* 1. No destructive changes on roentgenographic examination   2. Radiographic evidence of osteoporosis may be present
Stage II, Moderate

* 1. Radiographic evidence of osteoporosis, with or without slight subchondral bone destruction; slight cartilage destruction may be present
* 2. No joint deformities, although limitation of joint mobility may be present
  3. Adjacent muscle atrophy
  4. Extra-articular soft-tissue lesions such as nodules and tenosynovitis may be present

Stage III, Severe

* 1. Radiographic evidence of cartilage and bone destruction, in addition to osteoporosis
* 2. Joint deformity, such as subluxation, ulnar deviation, or hyperextension, without fibrous or bony ankylosis
  3. Extensive muscle atrophy
  4. Extra-articular soft-tissue lesions, such as nodules and tenosynovitis, may be present

Stage IV, Terminal
* 1. Fibrous or bony ankylosis   2. Criteria of stage III

* The criteria prefaced by an asterisk are those that must be present to permit classification of a patient in any particular stage or grade.

Reprinted from Steinbrocker O, Traeger CH, Batterman RC. Therapeutic criteria in rheumatoid arthritis. JAMA 1949; 140: 659–662, with permission of the American Medical Association.

Treatment

- **Goals** – The major goals of therapy are to relieve pain, swelling, and fatigue; improve joint function; halt joint damage; and prevent disability and disease-related morbidity.

- **Educate** – Patient education is essential early and throughout the disease course.

- **Referral** – Patients are served most effectively by a multidisciplinary approach that involves early referral to a rheumatologist who coordinates care with other health-care professionals, including nurses, occupational and physical therapists, and orthopedists.

- **Nonsteroidal anti-inflammatory drugs (NSAIDS)** – These, including COX-2 inhibitors, act quickly to reduce inflammation and pain but do not prevent tissue injury or progressive joint damage.

- **Glucocorticoids** – Low-dose glucocorticoids are potent suppressors of inflammation, and they are effective in managing the pain and functional limitations of people with active inflammatory joint disease.

- **Disease-modifying antirheumatic drugs (DMARDs) and biologic response modifiers** – An effective DMARD should control the active synovitis and constitutional features of the disease, thereby preventing joint erosions and damage. DMARDs do not heal erosions or reverse joint deformities. The ideal time to use a DMARD is early in the course of aggressive disease, before the appearance of erosive changes on radiographs. See the chapters on Therapies for information on specific drugs and appropriate monitoring.

American College of Rheumatology Preliminary Definition of Improvement in Rheumatoid Arthritis (ACR-20)

Required:	≥20% improvement in tender joint count ≥20% improvement in swollen joint count
Plus:	≥20% improvement in three of the following five: Patient gain assessment Patient global assessment Physician global assessment Patient self-assessed disability Acute-phase reactant (ESR or CRP)
Disease activity measure	**Method of assessment**
1. Tender joint count	ACR tender joint count, an assessment of 28 or more joints. The joint count should be done by scoring several different aspects of tenderness, as assessed by pressure and joint manipulation on physical examination. The information on various types of tenderness should then be collapsed into a single tender-versus-nontender dichotomy
2. Swollen joint count	ACR swollen joint count, an assessment of 28 or more joints. Joints are classified as either swollen or not swollen
3. Patient's assessment of pain	A horizontal, visual, analog scale (usually 10 cm) or Likert scale assessment of the patient's current level of pain
4. Patient's global assessment of disease activity	The patient's overall assessment of how the arthritis is doing. One acceptable method for determining this is the question from the AIMS instrument: "Considering all the ways your arthritis affects you, mark "X" on the scale for how well you are doing." An anchored, horizontal, visual, analog scale (usually 10 cm) should be provided. A Likert scale response is also acceptable
5. Physician's global assessment	A horizontal, visual, analog scale (usually 10 cm) or Likert scale measure of the physician's assessment of the patient's current disease activity
6. Patient's assessment of physical function	Any patient self-assessment instrument which has been validated, has reliability, has been proven in RA trials to be sensitive to change, and measures physical function in RA patients is acceptable. Instruments which have been demonstrated to be sensitive in RA trials include the AIMS, the HAQ, the Quality (or Index) of Well-Being, the MHIQ, and the MACTAR
7. Acute-phase reactant value	A Westergren ESR or a CRP level

ACR, American College of Rheumatology; AIMS, Arthritis Impact Measurement Scales; CRP, C-reactive protein; ESR, erythrocyte sedimentation rate; HAQ, Health Assessment Questionnaire; MACTAR, McMaster Toronto Arthritis Patient Preference Disability Questionnaire; MHIQ, McMaster Health Index Questionnaire; RA, rheumatoid arthritis.

Reprinted from Felson DT, Anderson JJ, Boers M, et al. American College of Rheumatology preliminary definition of improvement in rheumatoid arthritis. Arthritis Rheum 1995; 38: 727–735. Copyright © 1995 American College of Rheumatology. Reproduced with permission of John Wiley & Sons, Inc.

10 JUVENILE IDIOPATHIC ARTHRITIS

Juvenile idiopathic arthritis (JIA) is the most common form of childhood arthritis. JIA is an umbrella term for a group of conditions that have in common chronic arthritis. The disorder is subdivided into seven categories: systemic, oligoarthritis (subcategories of persistent and extended), polyarthritis rheumatoid factor (RF) positive, polyarthritis RF negative, enthesitis-related arthritis, psoriatic arthritis, and undifferentiated arthritis.

Clinical Features

- **Onset** – Before the age of 16 years.

- **Persistent objective arthritis** – Swelling, effusion, or the presence of two or more of the following – limitation of motion, tenderness, pain on motion, or joint warmth in one or more joints for at least six weeks. Exclusion of other causes of childhood arthritis.

- **Systemic JIA (sJIA)** – Growth delay, osteopenia, diffuse lymphadenopathy, hepatosplenomegaly, pericarditis, and pleuritis. Positive RF and uveitis are rare in this subset. Striking fevers with daily occurrence are typical of sJIA. Also characteristic is a fleeting, salmon-colored rash, which frequently develops with the fevers. Most systemic features resolve when the fevers subside; however, sJIA patients can develop pericardial tamponade, severe vasculitis with secondary consumptive coagulopathy, and macrophage activation syndrome. Most cases of sJIA start at 1–6 years of age. Boys and girls are affected equally.

- **Oligoarthritis** – JIA patients with oligoarthritis, sometimes said to have pauciarticular JIA, are divided into two subcategories: persistent and extended. Persistent oligoarthritis often has mild symptoms and the best overall articular outcome of all JIA categories. Up to 50% of oligoarthritis cases evolve to the extended subcategory. Compared with other subtypes, JIA patients with oligoarthritis are commonly younger (1–5 years at onset), more likely to be girls than boys (ratio 4:1), often antinuclear antibody (ANA) positive, and have the greatest risk for developing chronic eye inflammation.

- **Polyarthritis RF positive or negative** – RF+ patients are almost always girls with later-onset disease (≥8 years old). Symmetrical small joint arthritis is the rule rather than the exception in RF+ patients. The RF+ polyarthritis subtype shares human leukocyte antigen (HLA) associations with adult rheumatoid arthritis (RA). Compared with RF-negative children, JIA patients with polyarthritis who are RF+ are at greater risk for joint erosions, nodules, and poor functional outcomes, and are more likely to resemble adult-onset RA than any other JIA subset. Clinical manifestations of the polyarthritis form of JIA are highly variable, and include fatigue, anorexia, protein–calorie malnutrition, anemia, growth retardation, delay in sexual maturation, and osteopenia. Girls with JIA and polyarthritis outnumber boys (3:1).

- **Enthesitis-related arthritis (ERA)** – Inflammation at sites of tendinous/ligamentous attachments to bone and of joint capsule or fascia into bone. Patients with ERA may have extra-articular involvement including inflammatory bowel disease, acute uveitis and aortic valve insufficiency. Peripheral arthritis is more common in ERA than sacroiliac or lumbar spine involvement. Most patients will have four or more joints affected. ERA often develops into a condition readily identified as juvenile spondyloarthropathy, akin to a pediatric variant of ankylosing spondylitis.

- **Psoriatic arthritis** – Patients exhibiting signs of chronic arthritis in association with psoriasis with an onset ≤16 years are said to have psoriatic JIA. However, the classic psoriatic rash may not appear for many years after the onset of the arthritis. Typically, the arthritis is peripheral, asymmetric, and often involves the knees, ankles, and small joints of the hands and feet. At onset, ~70% of psoriatic JIA patients have arthritis in four or more joints. Involvement of the sacroiliac joint and asymptomatic chronic anterior chamber uveitis may develop.

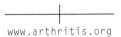

www.arthritis.org

- **Ocular involvement** – Chronic uveitis occurs most frequently in the oligoarthritis and psoriatic arthritis variants of JIA. On rare occasions, uveitis is reported in sJIA and in the polyarthritis variant. Chronic uveitis remains subclinical even while causing substantial ocular damage. Careful ophthalmologic examination and close follow-up are required.

Laboratory Features

- **Systemic** – Very high level of C-reactive protein (CRP), high erythrocyte sedimentation rate (ESR), neutrophilia, thrombocytosis, and hypochromic microcytic anemia. No serum autoantibodies or RF are detectable. Complement levels are normal or high. Immunologic abnormalities include the presence of polyclonal hypergammaglobulinemia, and elevated proinflammatory cytokines and chemokines.

- **Oligoarthritis** – In more severe/extended oligoarthritis, ESR and CRP are raised. RF is not present, but low-titer ANAs often are.

- **Polyarthritis** – RF+ patients also tend to have circulating anticyclic citrullinated peptide antibodies. RF-negative JIA is often associated with a positive test for ANAs.

Diagnosis

- **Combined approach** – Diagnosis requires a combination of data from history, physical examination and laboratory testing.

- **JIA** – Disease onset before the 16th birthday, persistent objective arthritis in one or more joints for at least six weeks, and exclusion of other causes of childhood arthritis.

- **Misdiagnosis** – Occurs when one or more of the following four key points are missed:

  1. Objective arthritis must be present. This is defined as joint swelling, joint effusion, or the presence of two or more of the following: limitation of motion, tenderness, pain on motion, or joint warmth. Arthralgias alone are not sufficient for the diagnosis of JIA.

  2. Arthritis must be consistently present for at least six weeks.

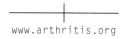

www.arthritis.org

3. Other causes of chronic arthritis in children must be excluded.

4. No specific laboratory or other test can establish the diagnosis of JIA; thus, it is a diagnosis of exclusion.

Treatment

- **Multidisciplinary approach** – Pediatric rheumatologists, ophthalmologists, orthopedic surgeons, dentists, physical and occupational therapists, dietitians, social workers, psychologists, and educational and vocational counselors.

- **Nonsteroidal anti-inflammatory drugs (NSAIDs)** – A four to six week trial is often required to assess effectiveness. Mostly used to alleviate pain, stiffness, and fever in sJIA.

- **Glucocorticoids** – Their negative impact on growth and bone limit their use in JIA. Systemic glucocorticoids are used mostly for uncontrolled fever, serositis, and the macrophage-activation syndrome in sJIA. They can also be used as a bridging medication while awaiting the effects of slower-acting agents. Intra-articular glucocorticoid injections are often highly effective in JIA.

Clinical Features of Each Juvenile Idiopathic

Classification
Systemic
Oligoarthritis (persistent)
Oligoarthritis (extended)
Polyarthritis RF+
Polyarthritis RF–
Enthesitis-related arthritis
Psoriatic arthritis
Undifferentiated

RF, rheumatoid factor; HLA, human leukocyte antigen.

ic Arthritis (JIA) Category

Description	Exclusions	Proportion of JIA population
Arthritis with or preceded by daily fever for ≥2 weeks, documented to be quotidian for ≥3 days, and accompanied by ≥1 of the following: transient, salmon-colored rash, generalized lymphadenopathy, hepato- or splenomegaly, and serositis	A, B, C, D	2–17%
Arthritis in ≤4 joints at any time during the onset or course of the disease	A, B, C, D, E	12–29%
Arthritis in ≤4 joints in first 6 months of disease but affecting a cumulative total of ≥5 joints after the first 6 months	A, B, C, D, E	12–29%
Arthritis affecting ≥5 joints after the first 6 months and positive test for RF at least twice ≥3 months apart	A, B, C, E	2–10%
Arthritis affecting ≥5 joints after the first 6 months with negative tests for RF	A, B, C, D, E	10–28%
Arthritis and enthesitis, or arthritis or enthesitis plus any 2 of the following: Sacroiliac joint tenderness and/or inflammatory lumbosacral pain Positive HLA-B27 Physician-diagnosed association with HLA-B27 in first- or second-degree relative Symptomatic anterior uveitis Male >6 years old at onset of arthritis or enthesitis	A, D, E	3–11%
Arthritis and psoriasis, or arthritis and ≥2 of the following: Physician-diagnosed psoriasis in first-degree relatives Dactylitis Nail abnormalities (pitting or onycholysis)	B, C, D, E	2–11%
Arthritis but does not fulfill any of the above categories or fits into more than one category	N/A	2–23%

Exclusion criteria:
A: Psoriasis in the patient or a first-degree relative.
B: Arthritis in a male positive for HLA-B27 with arthritis onset after 6 years of age.
C: Anklyosing spondylitis, enthesitis-related arthritis, sacroiliitis with inflammatory bowel disease, reactive arthritis, or acute anterior uveitis in a first-degree relative.
D: Presence of immunoglobulin (Ig)M RF on at least two occasions more than 3 months apart.
E: Presence of systemic JIA in the patient.
Data from Petty RE, et al. J Rheumatol 2004; 31: 390–392.

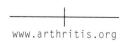

- **Methotrexate** – Cornerstone therapy for JIA. Efficacy varies in the subtypes of JIA. The greatest benefit is seen in patients with extended oligoarthritis. Methotrexate is less effective in sJIA.

- **Tumor necrosis factor (TNF) inhibitors** – Highly effective in polyarthritis, including patients who have failed methotrexate therapy. Less effective in sJIA. Screening for tuberculosis is required before TNF inhibitor use.

- **Other biologic response modifiers** – Anakinra, an inhibitor of IL-1, is often effective in treating cases of sJIA that are refractory to glucocorticoids and methotrexate, and is typically more effective than TNF inhibitors for this indication. Anakinra is less effective than anti-TNF medications in the treatment of polyarthritis. IL6 inhibition by tocilizumab appears to be a highly effective therapy for some variants of JIA. Studies of abatacept and rituximab in JIA are ongoing.

- **Ocular inflammation** – Treatment of uveitis should be directed by an ophthalmologist experienced in treating inflammatory eye disorders, with the guidance of pediatric rheumatologists experienced in managing immunosuppressive and biologic-modifying medications.

Special Considerations

Examination

- **Height and weight** – Should be obtained at each visit and plotted on an appropriate growth chart. Inadequately controlled disease or medication side effects can impair normal growth.

- **Infants and toddlers** – Observation skills are particularly important. Swelling can be subtle in a larger child and careful attention to range of motion is critical.

- **School-aged children** – Often like to participate in the examination. Careful attention should be paid to gait, leg length and muscle strength in addition to joint examination.

- **Adolescents** – The examination itself is not difficult but relating to the patient can be. Should include a scoliosis screen as part of the musculoskeletal examination.

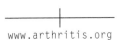

Growth

- **Multifactorial** – Growth impairment in JIA can result from the disease itself, in addition to medication side effects, nutritional and mechanical problems.

- **Impact of JIA subtype** – Little or no general adverse effect on growth in children with the oligoarthritis subtype. Polyarticular or systemic subtypes may retard growth, particularly in severe or long-standing disease.

- **Local impact** – Local growth disturbances occur as a result of inflammation and the accompanying increase in vascularity. This may result in either increased or diminished growth of the affected bone.

- **Other factors** – JIA patients are at risk for osteopenia and osteoporosis. Reduced serum levels of hormones essential for normal growth are common. Comorbid thyroid dysfunction may occur.

- **Nutrition** – Nutrition adequate in both calories and protein is critical to optimize growth.

Adherence

- **Factors affecting adherence** – These can generally be grouped into three categories: factors relating to the disease; factors relating to the patient and family; and those relating to the regimen itself.

- **Strategies for improving adherence** – Education, good organization, behavioral strategies, and anticipation of some of the known negative factors.

Child Development

- **Psychosocial** – Positive family factors may play an important role in the child's ability to cope with chronic illness.

- **School and educational achievement** – School success is critical to the normal development of the child, and school status and educational progress should be assessed regularly at clinic visits.

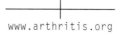

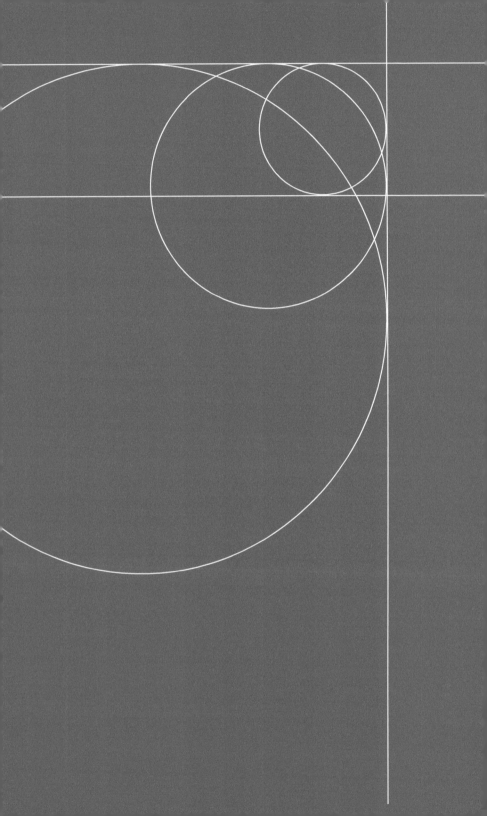

11 PSORIATIC ARTHRITIS

Psoriatic arthritis is a disease distinct from other inflammatory arthritides. It has features typical of the spondyloarthropathies in some patients, features of rheumatoid arthritis in others, and features of both in yet others.

Clinical Features

- **Three general types** – Monarthritis or oligoarthritis with enthesitis resembling reactive arthritis (30% to 50% of patients); symmetric polyarthritis resembling rheumatoid arthritis (30% to 50% of patients); and axial disease with or without peripheral joint disease (5% of patients).

- **Arthritis onset** – About 70% of patients have psoriasis many years before onset of arthritis.

- **Initial manifestation** – A mono- or oligoarticular arthritis, similar to the peripheral arthritis seen in the spondyloarthropathies, is observed in up to two-thirds of patients. A classic presentation includes oligoarticular arthritis involving a large joint (typically a knee or ankle), one or two interphalangeal joints (most often distal interphalangeal joints), and a dactylitic digit. In one-third to one-half of patients, oligoarthritis will evolve to a more symmetric polyarthritis that closely resembles RA.

- **Pattern of arthritis** – Symmetric polyarthritis involving the small joints of the hands and feet, wrists, ankles, knees, and elbows is the most common pattern of psoriatic arthritis.

- **Arthritis mutilans** – A rare, but highly destructive form of psoriatic arthritis affecting the digits.

- **Axial disease** – Axial arthritis may involve the sacroiliac joints as well as all segments of the spine.

- **Skin lesions** – The typical psoriatic skin lesion is a sharply demarcated erythematous plaque with a well-marked, silvery scale.

- **Nail involvement** – The only clinical feature that identifies patients with psoriasis who are likely to develop arthritis. Clinical signs include pitting, onycholysis, transverse depression and cracking, subungual keratosis, brown-yellow discoloration, and leukonychia.

Radiographic Features

- **Characteristic changes** – Marginal erosions, cartilage loss, and new bone formation.

Diagnosis

- **Exclude rheumatoid arthritis** – Features to distinguish psoriatic arthritis from RA: the presence of dactylitis and enthesitis, signs of psoriatic skin or nail disease, involvement of the distal interphalangeal joints, and the presence of spinal or sacroiliitis disease.

- **Exclude ankylosing spondylitis** – Features to distinguish psoriatic arthritis from ankylosing spondylitis: spine disease is less severe and appears at a later age in psoriatic arthritis, psoriatic skin or nail disease, family history of psoriasis, and less symmetric radiographic features.

- **Exclude reactive arthritis** – Features to distinguish psoriatic arthritis from reactive arthritis: lack of preceding infectious episode, predilection for joints of the upper extremities, and the absence of balanitis, urethritis, oral ulcers, and conjunctivitis.

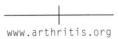

Treatment

- **Skin disease** – Topical application of emollients and keratolytic agents, alone or in combination with anthralin, glucocorticoids, vitamin D derivatives, and topical retinoids, help treat skin disease. Patients with extensive skin disease may benefit from photochemotherapy (PUVA) under the care of a dermatologist.

- **Joint disease** – Management follows the general principles of managing RA and the spondyloarthropathies.

- **NSAIDs** – NSAIDs are effective in most patients and should be the initial therapy for people with mild joint disease.

- **DMARDs** – DMARDs should be initiated as early as possible for patients whose conditions don't respond adequately to NSAIDs, and those who have progressive, erosive, polyarticular disease or oligoarticular disease involving large joints that does not respond to local glucocorticoid injections.

- **Methotrexate** – Methotrexate is effective for both the skin disease and peripheral arthritis in patients with oligo- or polyarticular disease.

- **Sulfasalazine** – Sulfasalazine is helpful for peripheral arthritis but not for axial disease, and it has no significant effect on the skin disease.

- **Glucocorticoids** – Steroids can be used safely in low doses, either in combination with DMARDs or as a bridge therapy while waiting for onset of action of DMARDs.

- **Biologic agents** – Tumor necrosis factor inhibitors should be considered in patients who fail to respond to DMARDs, and are effective for both arthritis and skin disease.

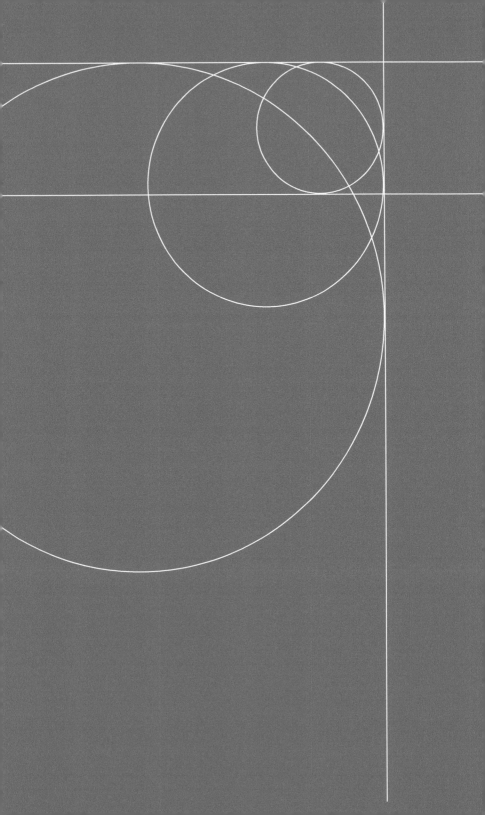

12 ANKYLOSING SPONDYLITIS

Ankylosing spondylitis (AS) is a chronic inflammatory disease of the sacroiliac joints and spine that may be associated with a variety of extraspinal lesions involving the eye, bowel, and heart.

Clinical Features

- **Presenting symptoms** – Insidious back pain with inflammatory features (e.g., morning stiffness), persistent for more than three months and worsened by rest but improved by exercise.

- **Constitutional features** – Fatigue, fever, and weight loss.

- **Age of onset** – Spinal features of AS seldom appear before the age of 18 years. The average age at the onset of clinical symptoms is 26 years. Earlier symptoms are often mild, ignored, or not recognized as AS. Thus, diagnostic delay is common.

- **Enthesitis** – A central feature of AS. In the spine, inflammation occurs at capsular and ligamentous attachments and discovertebral, costovertebral, and costotransverse joints, with involvement also at bony attachments of interspinous and paravertebral ligaments. Extraspinal enthesitis, e.g., at the Achilles tendon insertion into the heel, is common.

- **Sacroiliitis** – The most common feature of AS, which develops in late teens or the third decade of life. Causes lower back pain and pain in the buttocks, which typically alternates between left and right sides. Radiological involvement is usually symmetrical.

- **Synovitis** – Peripheral joint synovitis is typically oligoarticular, often asymmetric, and frequently episodic rather than persistent, in contrast to rheumatoid arthritis. Hips, knees, ankles, and metatarsophalangeal joints are affected most commonly. Upper limb joints are seldom involved, with the occasional exception of the shoulder.

- **Eye lesions** – Acute anterior uveitis (iritis) often develops at some time in about one-third of patients. Its occurrence is independent of arthritis flares.

- **Inflammatory bowel disease (IBD)** – Sacroiliitis occurs in up to 25% of people with IBD. In that setting, the activities of joint and bowel inflammation may not synchronize.

- **Less common organ involvement** – Aortic regurgitation, pulmonary fibrosis, and neurologic lesions following spinal fracture are other complications of AS.

Laboratory Features

- **Human leukocyte antigen (HLA)-B27** – A strong genetic risk factor for AS: present in >90% of patients with AS. However, this gene is neither necessary nor sufficient to cause the disease.

- **Seronegativity** – Absence of serum rheumatoid factor and antinuclear antibodies.

Imaging

- **Radiographic** – Inflammation of the spine and axial joints is a key characteristic. However, about 30% of the patients do not develop radiographic evidence of damage to the spine. Characteristic features on radiographs of the sacroiliac joints are pseudo-widening of the joint space, sclerosis, erosions and ankylosis, and progression to fusion. Changes in the spine include squaring of the vertebrae, sclerosis, erosions, syndesmophytes, bony bridging, and spondylodiscitis.

- **Magnetic resonance imaging (MRI)** – MRI of the sacroiliac joints and spine may be useful in cases of suspected AS when radiographs appear persistently normal. Unlike conventional radiographs, MRI has the potential to demonstrate inflammation and is useful in visualizing enthesitis.

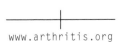

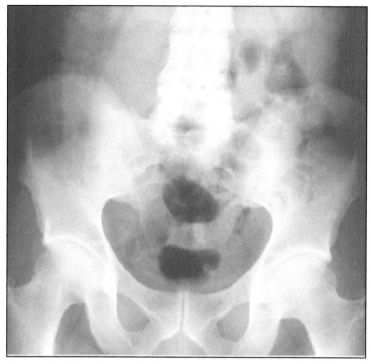

Anteroposterior radiographs of the pelvis showing complete ankylosis of both sacroiliac joints and syndesmophyte formation in the lower lumbar vertebrae.

Diagnosis

- **Combined approach** – The diagnosis rests on the combination of clinical features, radiological findings, laboratory results, and response to treatment.

- **HLA-B27** – When moderate to high suspicion of AS exists, presence of the HLA-B27 enhances the likelihood of AS.

- **Early diagnosis** – MRI confirmation of inflammation prior to the occurrence of radiographic evidence of joint damage may contribute to earlier diagnosis.

Modified New York Criteria Used for Diagnosis in Established Disease

Criteria	
1.	Low back pain for at least 3 months' duration improved by exercise and not relieved by rest
2.	Limitation of lumbar spine motion in sagittal and frontal planes
3.	Chest expansion decreased relative to normal values for age and sex
4a.	Unilateral sacroiliitis grade 3–4
4b.	Bilateral sacroiliitis grade 2–4
Definite ankylosing spondylitis if (4a OR 4b) AND any clinical criterion (1–3)	

Adapted with permission from Van der Linden et al. Arthritis Rheum 1984; 27: 361–368. Copyright © 1984 American College of Rheumatology. Reproduced with permission of John Wiley & Sons, Inc.

Amor's Classification for Spondyloarthritis in Atypical and Undifferentiated Cases

A	Clinical symptoms or history of	Scoring
1.	Lumbar or dorsal pain at night or morning stiffness of lumbar or dorsal pain	1
2.	Asymmetrical oligoarthritis	2
3.	Buttock pain	1
	If alternate buttock pain	2
4.	Sausage-like toe or digit	2
5.	Heel pain or other well-defined enthesopathy	2
6.	Iritis	1
7.	Nongonococcal urethritis or cervicitis within 1 month before the onset of arthritis	1
8.	Acute diarrhea within 1 month before the onset of arthritis	1
9.	Psoriasis, balanitis, or IBD (ulcerative colitis or Crohn's disease)	2
B	**Radiological findings**	
10.	Sacroiliitis (bilateral grade 2 or unilateral grade 3)	3
C	**Genetic background**	
11.	Presence of HLA-B27 and/or family history of ankylosing spondylitis, reactive arthritis, uveitis, psoriasis, or IBD	2
D	**Response to treatment**	
12.	Clear-cut improvement within 48 hours after nonsteroidal anti-inflammatory drugs (NSAIDs) intake or rapid relapse of the pain after their discontinuation	2

A patient is considered as suffering from a spondyloarthropathy if the sum is ≥6.
Adapted from: Amor B et al. [criteria of the classification of spondyloarthropathies.] Rev Rheum Mal Ostéoart. 1990; 57: 85–89. Copyright © 1990 Elsevier.

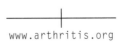

Treatment

- **Goals** – Symptom relief and the maintenance of function are the first goals of therapy. Major clinical responses and potentially disease-modifying benefits are possible through combined approaches to therapy.

- **Monitoring of disease activity** – Measurements of physical function, pain, spinal mobility, patient's global assessment, duration of morning stiffness, involvement of peripheral joints and entheses, acute-phase reactants, and fatigue. A physician's global assessment, taking into account available clinical, laboratory, and imaging data, should be performed.

- **Exercise** – Physical therapy, exercise, and patient education are the cornerstone of therapy and complement pharmacological therapies. Extended periods of immobility should be avoided.

- **Breathing** – Patients should be taught deep-breathing techniques and avoid smoking.

- **NSAIDs** – First-line therapy for AS. Symptomatic patients should be given a trial of at least two NSAIDs. Additional therapy should be given to patients with moderate disease activity or greater.

- **Muscle relaxants** – May alleviate stiffness.

- **Glucocorticoids** – Intra-articular injections may be helpful for peripheral arthritis. However, systemic glucocorticoids have little role. Glucocorticoid eye drops combined with a mydriatic agent are essential to the treatment of anterior uveitis.

- **Tumor necrosis factor (TNF) inhibitors** – TNF inhibitors are now the treatment of choice for patients with inadequate symptom relief from NSAIDs. All TNF inhibitors are effective for the articular manifestations of AS. Etanercept is not effective for the gastrointestinal manifestations of patients with IBD.

- **Surgical intervention** – Total hip arthroplasty, osteotomy, and fixation may greatly improve mobility and quality of life in properly selected patients.

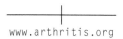

www.arthritis.org

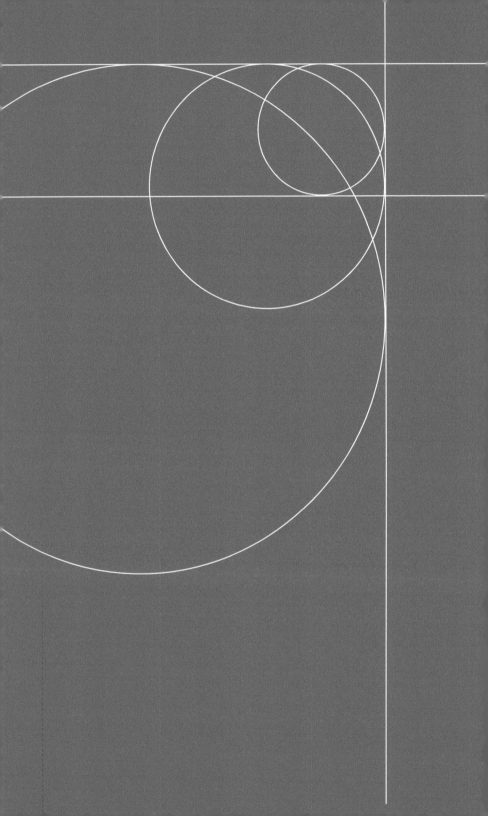

13 REACTIVE AND ENTEROPATHIC ARTHRITIS

Reactive Arthritis

Reactive arthritis (ReA) is a form of arthritis that occurs following exposure to infectious agents.

Clinical Features

- **Antecedent extra-articular infection** – Predominant organisms include *Chlamydia*, *Salmonella*, *Shigella*, *Yersinia*, and *Campylobacter* species.

- **Joints affected** – ReA is an oligoarthritic condition that characteristically affects the lower extremities in an asymmetric manner. Hip and upper extremity involvement without lower extremity disease is uncommon.

- **Signs and symptoms** – Joints are typically warm, swollen, and tender, and can mimic a septic arthritis.

- **Dactylitis (sausage digit)** – The involvement of all joints on a single finger, leading to the appearance of the digit as a sausage, is typical of ReA.

- **Enthesitis** – Achilles tendinitis and plantar fasciitis are common. Pain in the iliac crests, ischial tuberosities, and back may also occur.

- **Lower back and buttock pain** – Reflects sacroiliac joint inflammation and occurs in up to 50% of cases.

- **Extra-articular features** – Keratoderma blenorrhagicum, nail dystrophy, circinate balanitis, dysuria and pyuria, oral ulcers on the hard palate or tongue, and acute anterior uveitis.

Laboratory Features

- **Seronegativity** – Absence of serum rheumatoid factor (RF), antibodies to cyclic citrullinated peptides, and antinuclear antibodies.

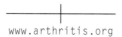

Diagnosis

- **Clinical diagnosis** – Presence of a seronegative, asymmetric oligoarthritis should alert a physician to the possibility of ReA. Previous infection and presence of common extra-articular manifestations associated with ReA provide further evidence. Symptoms of enthesitis, dactylitis, or mucocutaneous lesions increase the likelihood of ReA.

- **Exclude septic arthritis** – Aspiration of synovial fluid and cultures are mandatory to exclude active infection.

- **Exclude psoriatic arthritis** – Distal interphalangeal joint disease, pitting of nails, plaque-like lesions over elbows and knees are strongly supportive of psoriatic arthritis.

Treatment

- **Nonsteroidal anti-inflammatory drugs (NSAIDs)** – First-line therapy to control the acute synovitis and enthesitis.

- **Glucocorticoids** – Intra-articular glucocorticoid injections can be useful for relief in monarthritis.

- **Disease-modifying antirheumatic drugs (DMARDs)** – Second-line agents for persistent synovitis, particularly sulfasalazine and methotrexate.

- **Tumor necrosis factor (TNF) inhibitors** – TNF inhibitors are highly effective for spondyloarthropathies, including ReA.

Enteropathic Spondyloarthritis

Enteropathic arthritis is a spondyloarthritis associated with the inflammatory bowel diseases (IBDs: Crohn's disease and ulcerative colitis).

Clinical Features

- **IBD** – Enteropathic arthritis is more prevalent among patients with Crohn's disease than ulcerative colitis.

- **Arthritis** – Peripheral, axial, or mixed pattern. May precede the gastrointestinal (GI) symptoms, which is often regarded as undifferentiated spondyloarthritis until IBD symptoms become manifest.

- **Peripheral arthritis** – Typically pauciarticular and asymmetric, and may occur in a migratory pattern in some patients. Often nonerosive, flares are intermittent and can last up to six weeks. There is a predilection for lower extremity joints. Dactylitis and enthesitis reiterate the close relationship to the spondyloarthritis family. The activity of the peripheral arthritis generally correlates well with the degree of active bowel inflammation, particularly in ulcerative colitis.

- **Axial arthritis** – Indistinguishable clinically and radiographically from primary AS, although severity may be enhanced in IBD-related spondylitis.

- **Skin manifestations of IBD** – Skin lesions: erythema nodosum, which tends to mirror the activity of the bowel disease and can often parallel the activity of the peripheral arthritis. Pyoderma gangrenosum is less common. Crohn's disease may be associated with recurrent oral aphthous ulcers, which are difficult to distinguish from those of Behçet's syndrome.

- **Ocular complications of IBD** – Acute anterior uveitis follows the pattern characteristic of spondyloarthritis. Crohn's disease may also be associated with a chronic granulomatous uveitis.

Laboratory Features

- **Seronegativity** – RF, antibodies to cyclic citrullinated peptides, and antinuclear antibodies are generally absent.

- **Anemia** – Anemia of chronic disease and GI blood loss is common.

- **Acute-phase reactants** – C-reactive protein and erythrocyte sedimentation rate are often elevated when disease is active.

- **Human leukocyte antigen (HLA)-B27** – The axial form of IBD-related arthritis is associated with HLA-B27, although to a lesser extent than primary AS. The peripheral arthritis of IBD is not associated with HLA-B27.

Diagnosis

- **Clinical diagnosis** – Presence of a seronegative, pauciarticular and asymmetric arthritis or symptoms of AS with accompanying IBD should alert a physician to the possibility of enteropathic spondyloarthritis.

- **Magnetic resonance imaging (MRI)** – MRI is the most sensitive means for detecting sacroiliitis in IBD patients.

- **Radiographs** – Peripheral joints generally do not reveal erosive changes, but a destructive process can occur in the hip.

Treatment

- **NSAIDs** – First-line therapy to control the acute synovitis and enthesitis; however, they may exacerbate the underlying IBD and so should be used with caution.

- **Glucocorticoids** – Intra-articular glucocorticoid injections relieve exacerbations of peripheral arthritis. Budesonide is often used in Crohn's disease flares.

- **Sulfasalazine** – Effective in treating peripheral but not axial joint involvement.

- **TNF inhibitors** – Infliximab and adalimumab are effective in both peripheral and axial arthritis as well as the underlying bowel disease, particularly Crohn's disease. Etanercept helps control the arthritis but not the IBD aspect of the condition.

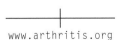

14 OSTEOARTHRITIS

Osteoarthritis is the most common form of arthritis. It is characterized by joint pain, tenderness, limitation of movement, crepitus, and variable degrees of local inflammation.

Clinical Features

- **Pain** – The cardinal symptom of OA, pain, is gradual onset, usually is mild to moderate in intensity, worsens by using the involved joints, and lessens or is relieved with rest. Initially, the pain may be intermittent, self-limited, and relieved by simple analgesics or nonsteroidal anti-inflammatory drugs (NSAIDs). With longer disease duration, the pain often becomes persistent.

- **Pain at rest** – Pain at rest or during the night is considered a feature of advanced disease.

- **Morning stiffness** – Common in people with OA, but the duration is shorter (often less than 30 minutes) than in rheumatoid arthritis. Gel phenomenon (stiffness after periods of rest and inactivity) is common in people with OA, but it resolves within several minutes.

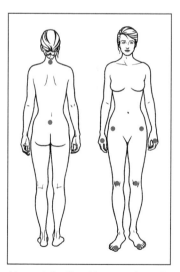

- **Changes in weather** – Pain and stiffness characteristically worsen in damp, cold, and rainy weather.

- **Joints affected** – Characteristic joints affected include knees, hips, lower spine, neck, feet, and hands.

Joints typically affected by osteoarthritis. The joints of the hand frequently affected are: the first carpometacarpal joint, the proximal interphalangeal joints, and the distal interphalangeal joints.

- **Knee OA** – Knee OA may be associated with instability or buckling, especially when descending stairs of stepping off curbs.

- **Hip OA** – Hip OA causes gait problems; pain is usually localized to the groin, and may radiate down the anterior thigh to the knee.

- **Hand OA** – Problems with manual dexterity, especially if there is involvement of the joints at the thumb base or the distal interphalangeal (DIP) joints.

- **Low back** – Diffuse pain across lower lumbar region, which can radiate into buttocks or posterior thigh.

- **Neck** – Pain in posterior cervical region, which can radiate to shoulders, suboccipital or interscapular areas, or to anterior chest.

- **Foot OA** – Most commonly involves big toe, causing the toe to move towards the outside of the foot (hallux valgus), and often a bunion forms.

- **Bony enlargement** – Bony enlargement is common, causing tenderness at the joint margins and at the attachments of the joint capsule and periarticular tendons.

- **Limitation of motion** – Loss of motion is usually related to osteophyte formation, severe cartilage loss leading to joint surface incongruity, or periarticular muscle spasm and contracture.

- **Periarticular muscle weakness** – Weakness is common and may contribute to progression of OA through decreased neuromuscular protective mechanisms and joint instability.

- **Joint instability** – Instability can be detected on physical examination by joint hypermobility.

- **Locking of a joint** – Joint locking is generally caused by loose bodies or floating cartilage fragments within the joint.

- **Crepitus** – Felt on passive range of motion, crepitus is due to irregularity of the opposing cartilage surfaces. This sign is common in people with OA of the knee.

- **Joint malalignment** – Almost 50% of patients with advanced knee OA have a malalignment of the joint, most commonly varus deformity due to loss of articular cartilage in the medial compartment.

- **Local inflammation** – Signs of inflammation include warmth and soft-tissue swelling due to joint effusion. However, the presence of a hot, erythematous, markedly swollen joint suggests either septic arthritis or a superimposed microcrystalline process, such as gout, pseudogout, or basic calcium phosphate (hydroxyapatite) arthritis.

Laboratory Features

- **Routine laboratory tests** – Normal.

- **Synovial fluid analysis** – Synovial fluid usually reveals a white blood cell (WBC) count below 2,000 cells/mm^3. The finding of inflammatory fluid with an elevated WBC count suggests either a superimposed microcrystalline process or septic arthritis.

Radiographic Features

- **Bony proliferation** – Osteophyte formation or spurs at the joint margin is the classic radiographic finding.

- **Asymmetric joint-space narrowing** – A decrease in interbone distance develops as the disease progresses.

- **Subchondral bone sclerosis** – Develops as the disease progresses.

- **Late changes** – Changes in the late disease include the formation of subchondral cysts with sclerotic walls and bone remodeling with alteration in the shape of bone ends.

- **Bone demineralization and marginal erosions** – Not radiographic features of OA.

Diagnosis

- **History and physical examination** – The diagnosis of OA almost always can be made by history and physical examination.

- **Identify characteristic pattern** – One or more of the following joint groups are affected in OA: distal interphalangeal, proximal interphalangeal, and first carpometacarpal joints of the hands; apophy-

Criteria for the Classification and Reporting of Osteoarthritis of the Hand, Hip, and Knee

Classification criteria for osteoarthritis of the hand[a]	Classification criteria for osteoarthritis of the hip, traditional format[b]
Hand pain, aching, or stiffness and Three or four of the following features: Hard tissue enlargement of two or more of 10 selected joints Hard tissue enlargement of two or more DIP joints Fewer than three swollen MCP joints Deformity of at least one of 10 selected joints	Hip pain and At least two of the following three features: ESR <20 mm/h Radiographic femoral or acetabular osteophytes Radiographic joint space narrowing (superior, axial, and/or medial)

a The 10 selected joints are the second and third distal interphalangeal (DIP), the second and third proximal interphalangeal, and the first carpometacarpal joints of both hands. This classification method yields a sensitivity of 94% and a specificity of 87%. DIP, distal interphalangeal; MCP, metacarpophalangeal.

Reprinted from Altman R, Alarcon G, Appelrouth D, et al. The American College of Rheumatology criteria for the classification and reporting of osteoarthritis of the hand. Arthritis Rheum 1990; 33: 1601–1610. Copyright © 1990 American College of Rheumatology. Reproduced with permission of John Wiley & Sons, Inc.

b This classification method yields a sensitivity of 89% and a specificity of 91%. ESR, erythrocyte sedimentation rate (Westergren).

Reprinted from Altman R, Alarcon G, Appelrouth D, et al. American College of Rheumatology criteria for the classification and reporting of osteoarthritis of the hip. Arthritis Rheum 1991; 34: 505–514. Copyright © 1991 American College of Rheumatology. Reproduced with permission of John Wiley & Sons, Inc.

Classification criteria for osteoarthritis of the knee[c]	
Clinical and laboratory	Clinical and radiographic
Knee pain plus at least five of nine: Age >50 years Stiffness <30 minutes Crepitus Bony tenderness Bony enlargement No palpable warmth ESR <40 mm/h RF <1:40 SF OA	Knee pain plus at least one of three: Age >50 years Stiffness <30 minutes Crepitus + Osteophytes
92% sensitive 75% specific	91% sensitive 86% specific

seal joints of the cervical and lumbar spine; first metatarsophalan-geal joints of the feet; knees; and hips. Involvement within a joint group usually is bilateral.

- **Exclude RA** – Generalized OA can be distinguished from rheu-matoid arthritis by the pattern of joint involvement in the hands; rheumatoid arthritis typically involves the metacarpophalangeal and proximal interphalangeal joints and wrists, but spares the thumb base and distal interphalangeal joints.

- **Exclude polymyalgia rheumatica** – People with OA of the axial skel-eton who have muscle aches in the neck, shoulder girdle, low back, and pelvic girdle should be evaluated for polymyalgia rheumatica.

- **Exclude underlying disorder** – People with OA involving atypical joints (e.g. metacarpophalangeal joints of the hands, wrists, elbows, shoulders, or ankles) should be evaluated for an underlying disor-der, such as calcium pyrophosphate dehydrate deposition disease or hemochromatosis.

- **Algorithms** – The American College of Rheumatology has developed algorithms for the classification of OA of the hands, hips, and knees.

Clinical[d]
Knee pain plus at least three of six:
Age >50 years
Stiffness <30 minutes
Crepitus
Bony tenderness
Bony enlargement
No palpable warmth
95% sensitive
69% specific

[c] ESR, erythrocyte sedimentation rate (Westergren); RF, rheumatoid factor; SF OA, synovial fluid signs of OA (clear, viscous, or white blood cell count <2,000/mm^3).

[d] Alternative for the clinical category would be four of six, which is 84% sensitive and 89% specific.

Reprinted from Altman R, Asch E, Bloch G et al. Development of the criteria for the classification and reporting of osteoarthritis: classification of osteoarthritis of the knee. Arthritis Rheum 1986; 29: 1039–1049. Copyright © 1986 American College of Rheumatology. Reproduced with permission of John Wiley & Sons, Inc.

Recommendations for the Medical Management of Osteoarthritis of the Hip and Knee

Nonpharmacologic therapy for patients with osteoarthritis
Patient education Self-management programs (e.g. Arthritis Foundation Self-Management Program) Personalized social support through telephone contact Weight loss (if overweight) Aerobic exercise programs Physical therapy Range-of-motion exercises Muscle-strengthening exercises Assistive devices for ambulation Patellar taping Appropriate footwear Lateral-wedged insoles (for genu varum) Bracing Occupational therapy Joint protection and energy conservation Assistive devices for activities of daily living
Pharmacologic therapy for patients with osteoarthritis[a]

Oral
    Acetaminophen
    COX-2 specific inhibitor
    Nonselective NSAID plus misoprostol or a proton pump inhibitor[b]
    Nonacetylated salicylate
    Other pure analgesics
        Tramadol
        Opioids
Intra-articular
    Glucocorticoids
    Hyaluronan
Topical
    Capsaicin
    Methylsalicylate

[a] The choice of agent(s) should be individualized for each patient. COX-2, cyclooxygenase 2; NSAID, nonsteroidal anti-inflammatory drug.

[b] Misoprostol and proton pump inhibitors are recommended in patients who are at increased risk for upper gastrointestinal adverse events.

Reprinted from American College of Rheumatology Subcommittee on Osteoarthritis Guidelines. Recommendations for the medical management of osteoarthritis of the hip and knee. Arthritis Rheum 2000; 43: 1905–1915. Copyright © 2000 American College of Rheumatology. Reproduced with permission of John Wiley & Sons, Inc.

- **Guidelines** – The American College of Rheumatology (ACR) has published guidelines for the medical management of OA of the hip and knee.

- **Alternative therapies** – Most popular supplements are glucosamine and chondroitin. See Chapter 36 for more information.

- **Surgery** – Patients with hip or knee OA whose symptoms are not controlled with other therapies and/or who have significant functional limitations are candidates for total joint replacement surgery.

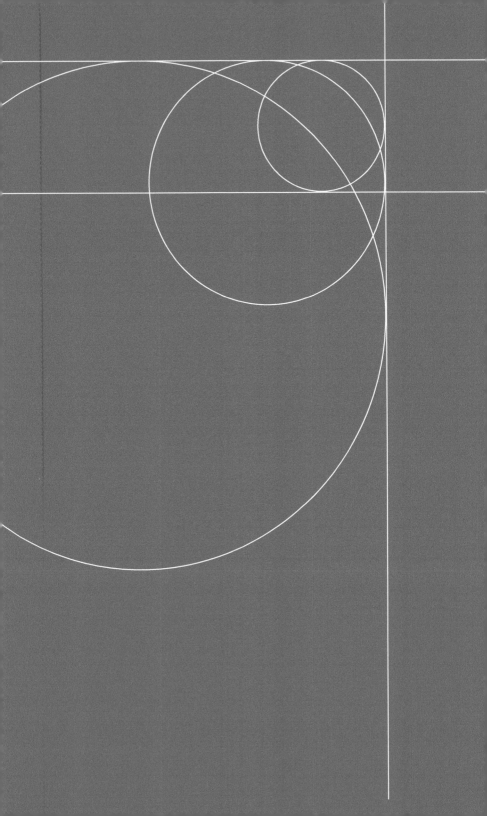

15 CALCIUM PYROPHOSPHATE DIHYDRATE, HYDROXYAPATITE, AND MISCELLANEOUS CRYSTALS

Calcium pyrophosphate dihydrate (CPPD) and hydroxyapatite crystals are the most common calcium-containing crystals associated with joint and periarticular disorders.

Calcium Pyrophosphate Dihydrate Crystals

Clinical Features

- **Crystal deposition** – The identification of CPPD crystals in synovial fluid or articular tissue allows differentiation between CPPD crystal deposition disease and other inflammatory and degenerative types of arthritis. CPPD crystals are sometimes deposited in synovial lining, ligaments, tendons, and, on rare occasions, periarticular soft tissue.

- **Pseudogout** – Acute, gout-like attacks of inflammation that occur with pain, stiffness, and swelling in the affected joint. Signs include swelling, variable degrees of erythema, and warmth. Compared with true gout, pseudogout attacks may take longer to reach peak intensity, and often last longer than gout attacks. Pseudogout is more common in large than small joints. Systemic manifestations during an attack may include significant fever (e.g., 102–103°F). About 25% of people with CPPD deposition exhibit the pseudogout pattern of disease.

- **Pseudo-osteoarthritis** – Gradual onset of joint pain and stiffness, typically involving knees, wrists, metacarpophalangeal joints, hips, shoulders, spine, elbows, and ankles. Most patients with clinically apparent CPPD crystal deposition have an unusually severe, oddly distributed, degenerative arthritis resembling osteoarthritis.

- **Pseudo-rheumatoid arthritis** – Multiple joint involvement with symmetric distribution and low-grade inflammation. This can be accompanied by morning stiffness, fatigue, synovial thickening, and flexion contractures.

- **Pseudo-neuropathic anthropathy** – Some patients with CPPD deposition disease have a severe destructive monarthritis similar to that seen in neuropathic joints.

- **Lanthanic** – Evidence of articular chondrocalcinosis – characteristic radiographic features of CPPD deposition in articular cartilage – with no clinically apparent arthritis.

Laboratory Features

- **Pseudogout** – Peripheral leukocytosis of 12,000–15,000 cells/mm^3 and elevated serum acute-phase reactants. Synovial fluid cell counts typically show white blood cell counts in the order of 30,000–75,000 cells/mm^3.

- **Pseudo-rheumatoid arthritis** – Elevated acute phase reactants; low rheumatoid factor titers in 10% of patients.

Diagnosis

- **Polarizing light microscopy** – Allows accurate identification of CPPD crystals in the synovial fluid of affected joints.

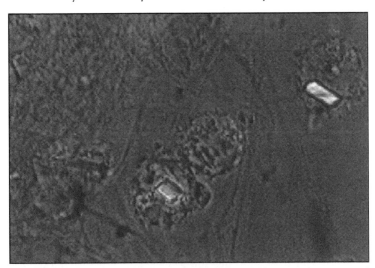

Rod-shaped calcium pyrophosphate dihydrate (CPPD) crystals in synovial fluid analyzed by compensated polarized light microscopy.

Diagnostic Criteria for CPPD Crystal Deposition Disease

Criteria
I.   Demonstration of CPPD crystals in tissue or synovial fluid by definitive means (e.g. characteristic X-ray diffraction or chemical analysis)
II. (a) Identification of monoclinic or triclinic crystals showing weakly positive or no birefringence by compensated polarized light microscopy
(b) Presence of typical radiographic calcification
III. (a) Acute arthritis, particularly of knees or other large joints
(b) Chronic arthritis, particularly of knee, hip, wrist, carpus, elbow, shoulder, or metacarpophalangeal joint, particularly if accompanied by acute exacerbations. The following features help differentiate chronic arthritis from osteoarthritis:
1. Uncommon site – wrist, metacarpophalangeal, elbow, and shoulder
2. Radiographic appearance – radiocarpal or patellofemoral joint space narrowing, particularly if isolated (patella "wrapped around" the femur)
3. Subchondral cyst formation
4. Severity of degeneration – progressive, with subchondral bony collapse and fragmentation with formation of intra-articular radiodense bodies
5. Osteophyte formation – variable and inconstant
6. Tendon calcifications, particularly triceps, Achilles, and obturators
Categories
A. Definite disease: Criteria I or II (a) plus II (b) must be fulfilled
B. Probable disease: Criteria II (a) or II (b) must be fulfilled
C. Possible disease: Criteria III (a) or III (b) should alert the clinician to the possibility of underlying CPPD crystal deposition

Radiographic Features

- **Punctate and linear densities** – These findings in articular hyaline or fibrocartilagenous tissues are helpful diagnostically. However, 50% of elderly individuals have radiographic evidence of CPPD, although most of those do not have pseudogout.

- **Screening views** – An individual can be screened for CPPD deposits with four radiographs: an anteroposterior (AP) view of both

knees (preferably not standing), an AP view of the pelvis for visualization of the symphysis pubis and hips, and a posteroanterior view
of both hands and wrists.

- **Metacarpophalangeal joints** – Squaring of the bone ends, subchondral cysts, and hook-like osteophytes are characteristic features of
the arthritis associated with hemochromatosis, but are also found
in patients with CPPD deposition alone.

Treatment

There is no practical way to remove CPPD crystals from joints; treatment is symptomatic.

- **Aspiration** – Acute attacks in large joints can be treated through
aspiration combined with injection of glucocorticoids.

- **Nonsteroidal anti-inflammatory drugs (NSAIDs)** – Recommended for most patients.

- **Oral colchicine** – Frequency and duration of acute attacks are
reduced significantly by colchicine taken on a daily basis for prophylaxis.

- **Systemic glucocorticoids** – Effective if multiple joints are involved
during the same pseudogout flare.

Apatite/Basic Calcium Phosphates

Basic calcium phosphate (BCP) crystals frequently deposit in articular
tissues.

Clinical Features

- **Osteoarthritis** – BCP crystals are present in 30–60% of patients
with knee osteoarthritis, but in many cases their presence remains
undetected.

- **Shoulder** – Typical patients are elderly women who manifest large,
noninflammatory synovial effusions, severe radiographic damage
and large rotator cuff tears. Patients typically have pain on shoulder

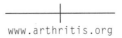

use and at night, with reduced active and passive range of motion, sometimes associated with pronounced joint instability.

- **Calcific periarthritis** – Calcification most commonly occurs in the rotator cuff tendons. This is accompanied by severe local pain, warmth, erythema, and joint swelling.

- **Acute arthritis** – In rare cases, BCP crystals may cause acute inflammation in joints.

- **Calcinosis** – Occurs in a wide variety of conditions. Idiopathic tumoral calcinosis is a rare syndrome characterized by the presence of irregular calcifying masses in periarticular soft tissue.

Diagnosis

- **Microscopy** – Polarized light microscopy is unable to detect BCP crystals because of their small size. Alizarin red S staining is used to help visualize the crystals.

Radiographic Features

- **Periarticular calcification** – Occasionally observed on shoulder or other radiographs.

- **Destructive arthritis of the shoulder** – Upward subluxation and deformity of the humeral head, and calcification of the tendinous rotator cuff.

Treatment

- **NSAIDs** – Commonly used to alleviate acute pain and inflammation.

Miscellaneous Crystals

- **Oxalate crystals** – Oxalates have been described in the joints of patients with overt renal failure only. Acute or chronic arthritis resulting from oxalate deposition occurs most frequently in the knees and hands.

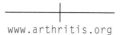

www.arthritis.org

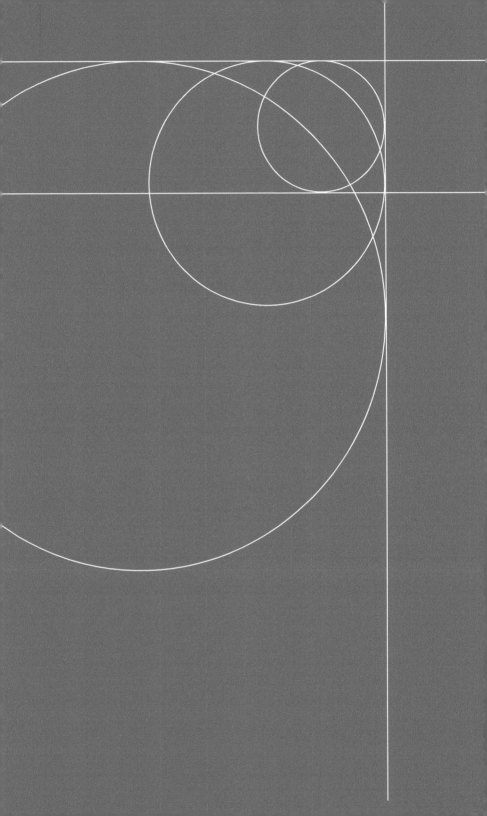

16 INFECTIOUS DISORDERS

Normal joints, joints affected with arthritis, and prosthetic joints are all vulnerable to infection.

Septic Arthritis

Clinical Features

- **Risk factors** – Age older than 80 years, diabetes mellitus, pre-existing rheumatoid arthritis, the presence of a prosthetic joint in the knee or hip, recent joint surgery, and skin infection.

- **Joints affected** – Septic arthritis is monarticular in 80–90% of cases and polyarticular in 10–20%. Large peripheral joints are infected more commonly than small ones.

- **Suspect septic arthritis** – Septic arthritis always is a consideration in a person presenting with an acute monarthritis, especially if the patient is febrile, appears toxic, or has an extra-articular site of bacterial infection.

- **Underlying inflammatory arthritis** – An acute exacerbation of joint inflammation, whether monarticular or polyarticular, must raise the suspicion of superimposed infection in a person with underlying inflammatory arthritis.

- **Gonococcal arthritis** – Most common form of septic arthritis in young, sexually active people. Typically a migratory pattern with prominent tenosynovitis and skin lesions.

- **Hepatitis B virus** – Arthritis onset is often sudden and severe.

- **Hepatitis C virus** – Triad of arthritis, palpable purpura, and (mixed) cryoglobulinemia.

- **HIV** – Several musculoskeletal syndromes described, including reactive arthritis and psoriatic arthritis.

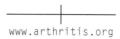

Laboratory Features

- **Synovial fluid** – The WBC range can vary widely from a few thousand cells to more than 100,000 cells/mm^3; typically, polymorphonuclear cells predominate (90% or greater).

- **Gram stain** – Smear of the infected synovial fluid is positive 60–80% of the time.

- **Culture** – Culture synovial fluid for microorganisms.

Diagnosis

- **Suspect septic arthritis** – Arthrocentesis is indicated, and the synovial fluid should be examined carefully for evidence of bacterial infection. If the synovial-fluid cell count is extremely high – e.g. 100,000 WBC per mm^3 or greater – treatment for presumed septic arthritis should be initiated, pending result of the fluid culture.

- **Pseudoseptic arthritis** – An extremely inflammatory arthritis not due to bacterial infection can be diagnosed only when one is confident that infectious causes have been excluded. The causes of pseudoseptic arthritis are listed. To confirm this diagnosis, a negative Gram stain or a negative culture of the synovial fluid should be corroborated by negative blood cultures.

Treatment

- **Prompt treatment** – Will eradicate infection, speed recovery, and decrease morbidity.

- **Begin antibiotics immediately** – If a presumptive diagnosis of septic arthritis has been made, and the appropriate samples for microbiologic studies have been collected, antibiotic treatment should begin immediately, even before the identity of the microorganism is known.

Conditions that may Present as Pseudoseptic Arthritis

Rheumatoid arthritis
Juvenile rheumatoid arthritis
Gout
Pseudogout
Apatite-related arthropathy
Reactive arthritis
Psoriatic arthritis
Systemic lupus erythematosus
Sickle cell disease
Dialysis-related amyloidosis
Transient synovitis of the hip
Plant thorn synovitis
Metastatic carcinoma
Pigmented villonodular synovitis
Hemarthrosis
Neuropathic arthropathy

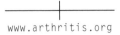

- **Antibiotic choice** – Initial choice depends on results of the Gram stain of the synovial fluid and the most likely causative organism. Antibiotic can be changed once culture and sensitivities are known.

- **Drain joint space** – The infected joint space must be completely drained initially, and then daily thereafter as long as fluid continues to reaccumulate.

- **Immobilization and analgesics** – During the initial few days, immobilization of the affected joint and effective analgesic medication will ensure patient comfort.

- **Physical therapy** – Should be instituted as soon as inflammation begins to subside and the patient can tolerate and undergo therapy.

Lyme Disease

Lyme disease is a multisystem inflammatory disease caused by the tick-borne spirochete *Borrelia burgdorferi*.

Clinical Features

- **Erythema migrans** – Rash occurs within one month of tick bite in 90% of patients. Most commonly found in or near the axilla, inguinal region, or belt line. One-half of patients with EM have multiple lesions.

- **Early localized disease** – Nonspecific complaints include fever, fatigue, malaise, headache, myalgias, and arthralgias. Physical examination occasionally reveals regional or generalized lymphadenopathy or hepatosplenomegaly.

- **Early disseminated disease** – Occurs days to months after the tick bite, and may occur without preceding EM. The two most common manifestations are cardiac and neurologic involvement. Cardiac manifestations include heart block and mild myopericarditis. Neurologic disease includes aseptic meningitis, cranial nerve palsies (most commonly Bell's palsy), and radiculoneuritis.

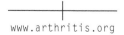

- **Late disease** – Occurs months to years after onset of infection, is not necessarily preceded by other features of Lyme disease, and most commonly involves arthritis and neurologic disease.

- **Chronic arthritis of Lyme disease** – Usually monarticular, and most commonly affects the knee. It occurs in approximately 10% of patients and can cause erosion of cartilage and bone.

- **Chronic neurologic manifestations** – Include encephalopathy, peripheral neuropathy, and cognitive dysfunction.

Laboratory Features

- **Antibodies to *Borrelia*** – An enzyme-linked immunosorbent assay (ELISA) is used to screen for antibodies to *Borrelia*. The current practice is to confirm all positive or equivocal ELISA results with Western blot analysis.

Diagnosis

- **History and physical findings** – The diagnosis of Lyme disease should be based on a history and objective physical findings explicitly suggesting the diagnosis.

- **Confirm** – Diagnosis by serologic testing.

- **False positive** –Individuals with positive ELISA not corroborated by Western blot are considered to have false-positive ELISA results. False-positive ELISA results occur in up to 5% of the population, and they have been reported in patients with other spirochetal infections (e.g. relapsing fever, syphilis, leptospirosis, etc.), Epstein-Barr virus infection, rheumatoid arthritis, and systemic lupus erythematosus.

- **Seropositive** – Most people with chronic manifestations are strongly seropositive, even if they have received antibiotics. Thus, seronegativity in patients with features indicative of late Lyme disease should raise doubts about the diagnosis.

- **Exclude similar entities** – Differentiate between four commonly confused entities: true infection (Lyme disease); post-Lyme disease syndromes; Lyme anxiety; and concurrent, unrelated medical occurrences. Post-Lyme disease syndromes occur in patients with prior, cured infection. Examples include fibromyalgia, sleep disorder, patellofemoral joint dysfunction, and poorly defined autoimmune phenomena.

Current Recommendations for Therapy in Lyme Disease

Drug	Dosage	Duration
Oral therapy of early localized Lyme disease		
Adults		
Doxycycline[a]	100 mg p.o., b.i.d.	3–4 weeks[d]
Tetracycline[a,b]	250–500 mg p.o., q.i.d.	3–4 weeks[d]
Amoxicillin[b,c]	250–500 mg p.o., q.i.d.	3–4 weeks[d]
Children		
Amoxicillin	40 mg/kg/day, divided dose	3–4 weeks[d]
Erythromycin	30 mg/kg/day, divided dose	3–4 weeks[d]
Penicillin G	25–50 mg/kg/day, divided dose	3–4 weeks[d]
Intravenous therapy of early disseminated and late Lyme disease[e]		
Adults		
Third-generation cephalosporins		
Ceftriaxone	2 g q.i.d. or 1 g b.i.d	2–4 weeks
Cefotaxime	3 g b.i.d.	2–4 weeks
Penicillin G	20 million U in 6 divided doses	4 weeks
Chloramphenicol	50 mg/kg/day in 4 divided doses	2–4 weeks
Children		
Third-generation cephalosporins		
Ceftriaxone	75–100 mg/kg/day	2–4 weeks
Cefotaxime	90–180 mg/kg/day in 2 or 3 divided doses	2–4 weeks
	300,000 U/kg/day in 6 divided doses	2–4 weeks
Penicillin G		

[a] No studies comparing doxycycline with tetracycline have been done.

[b] Dosage determined by weight of patient.

[c] No studies comparing amoxicillin with amoxicillin plus probenecid have been done; cefuroxime axetil and azithromycin have also been studied in Lyme disease.

[d] There is no proof that this is the optimal duration of therapy or that more than 10–14 days of treatment is necessary.

[e] There is no proof that isolated facial nerve palsy or carditis must be treated with intravenous therapy. Oral doxycycline for early Lyme neuroborreliosis has been shown to be effective in European studies. Especially in children, oral treatment for Lyme arthritis may suffice.

Adapted from Sigal LH. Current drug therapy recommendations for the treatment of Lyme disease. Drugs 1992; 43: 683–699, with permission of Wolters Kluwer Health.

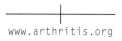

Treatment

- **Antibiotic treatment** – Treating *B. burgdorferi* infection in early disease usually prevents progression and is curative.

- **Refractory Lyme arthritis** – May benefit from intra-articular glucocorticoid injections, hydroxychloroquine, or synovectomy.

- **Response to therapy** – There may be persistent nonspecific complaints for many months following adequate treatment.

17 SYSTEMIC LUPUS ERYTHEMATOSUS

Systemic lupus erythematosus (SLE) is an inflammatory, autoimmune disorder that affects multiple organ systems, particularly the skin, joints, kidneys, and central nervous system.

Clinical Features

- **Constitutional features** – Fatigue, fever, and weight loss during disease flares.

Skin

- **Malar or "butterfly" rash** – The most classic lupus rash. An erythematous, edematous eruption that extends over the bridge of the nose and involves the malar eminences. The rash has texture (i.e., is not flat), but is non-scarring. May also be seen on the chin or forehead.

- **Discoid lupus (DLE)** – Discrete plaques, erythematous and scaling early in the disease, with progression to chronic scarring lesions. Commonly occur on face, ears, scalp, and trunk. Can occur as part of the systemic disease or in isolation.

- **Lupus panniculitis** – Rare. Painful inflammatory lesions involving the deep dermis and subcutaneous fat. Typically develop on buttocks, abdominal wall, and legs.

- **Subacute cutaneous lupus erythematosus (SCLE)** – The lesions begin as small, erythematous, scaly papules or plaques that can evolve into papulosquamous (psoriasiform) or annular polycyclic forms. Typically widespread, superficial, and non-scarring, and most often present in sun-exposed areas. Associated with antibodies to the Ro/SSA antigen.

- **Alopecia** – Has a variety of causes in SLE. May be diffuse or patchy, reversible or permanently scarring. May occur in a patchy fashion as a result of discoid lesions, in which case scarring usually develops. Can also develop more diffusely following a period of intense disease activity; in this case the hair returns following a return of disease quiescence. Also caused by numerous SLE medications.

- **Mucosal lesions** – Can affect the buccal mucosa and nose.

- **Vasculitis** – May manifest as palpable purpura, erythematous papules of the pulps of the fingers and palms, or splinter hemorrhages.

- **Vasculopathy** – Presents as nailfold or digital ulcerations (the "digital pitting" also described in scleroderma) or frank digital ischemia.

Musculoskeletal System

- **Arthritis, arthralgia** – Joint complaints ranging from pain without frank arthritis to swelling, erythema, tenderness, and decreased range of motion.

- **Joints affected** – Although arthritis can affect any joint, it is most often symmetric with involvement of the small joints of the hands (proximal interphalangeal and metacarpophalangeal), wrists, and knees, but sparing the spine. May be difficult to distinguish from other inflammatory arthropathies, particularly rheumatoid arthritis (RA).

- **Myalgia and muscle weakness** – Frequently involving the deltoids and quadriceps, can be accompanying features of disease flares. Muscle weakness may also occur as a result of glucocorticoid therapy (steroid myopathy).

Renal

- **Asymptomatic** – There are typically few signs or symptoms of renal disease until advanced stages. Edema or weight gain may be associated with nephrotic syndrome. Profound fatigue accompanies advanced renal dysfunction.

- **Abnormal urinalysis** – Renal disease typically first evident with abnormalities found on urinalysis including hematuria, sterile pyuria, cellular casts, and proteinuria.

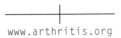

www.arthritis.org

- **Proteinuria** – Spot urine protein/creatinine ratios or 24-hour urine collections are helpful in quantifying proteinuria. The former are easier to obtain and should be estimated at each visit.

- **Renal function** – Assessed by a serum creatinine or blood urea nitrogen measurement, or estimation of creatinine clearance.

- **Renal biopsy** – Not required to diagnose lupus nephritis, but helpful in guiding treatment decisions and determining prognosis. Greatest likelihood of progressive renal dysfunction is associated with diffuse proliferative glomerulonephritis.

Nervous System

- **Neuropsychiatric systemic lupus** – Includes syndromes of the central, peripheral, and autonomic nervous systems.

- **Psychiatric disorders** – Include mood disorders, anxiety, and psychosis.

- **Cognitive defects** – Include attention deficit, poor concentration, impaired memory, difficulty in word finding, and acute confusional state.

- **Seizures** – May be focal or generalized.

- **Meningitis** – Aseptic meningitis can result from either SLE or as a complication of treatment with nonsteroidal anti-inflammatory drugs (NSAIDs).

- **Cranial nerves** – Disturbances of the cranial nerves can result in visual defects, blindness, papilledema, nystagmus or ptosis, tinnitus and vertigo, and facial palsy.

Cardiovascular System

- **Pericarditis** – Substernal or anterior chest pain, aggravated by motion, such as inspiration, coughing, swallowing, twisting, and bending forward. Echocardiogram helpful in detecting pericardial effusion.

- **Accelerated atherosclerosis** – An important cause of morbidity and mortality in SLE.

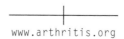

- **Primary myocardial involvement** – Uncommon (<5%). Signs include fever, dyspnea, palpitations, heart murmurs, sinus tachycardia, ventricular arrhythmias, conduction abnormalities, or congestive heart failure.

Pleura and Lungs

- **Pleuritis** – Common, with lateral chest or flank pain that increases with inspiration. Pleural effusions may develop and be detected on chest radiographs.

- **Pulmonary involvement** – Includes pneumonitis, pulmonary hemorrhage, pulmonary embolism, and shrinking-lung syndrome.

- **Pulmonary hypertension** – Should be suspected in patients complaining of progressive shortness of breath, and in whom the chest radiograph is negative and profound hypoxemia is absent.

Autoantibodies and Clinical Features

Antibodies (%)	Frequency
ANA	>90
Anti-dsDNA	40–60
Anti-RNP	30–40
Anti-ribosomal P	10–20
Anti-SSA/Ro	30–45
Anti-SSB/La	10–15
Antiphospholipid	30

ANA, antinuclear antibodies; dsDNA, double-stranded DNA; RNP, ribonucleoprotein; SCLE, subacute cutaneous lupus erythematosus.

Laboratory Features

Hematologic Abnormalities

- **CBC** – A complete blood count is a critical part of the initial and continued evaluation of all people with SLE because all cell lines can be affected.

- **Anemia** – Anemia of chronic disease (low-grade, common) or hemolytic (rare). Iron-deficiency anemia also occurs because many SLE patients are young women.

- **Leukopenia** – Either lymphopenia or neutropenia may be observed.

Clinical associations	Relationship to disease activity
Nonspecific	For diagnostic purposes only. Serial assessment not required once diagnosis established
Nephritis	Rough correlation with disease activity in some case
Raynaud's, musculoskeletal	Poor correlation
Diffuse CNS, psychosis, major depression	Poor correlation
Dry eyes and mouth, SCLE, neonatal lupus, photosensitivity	Poor correlation
Dry eyes and mouth, SCLE, neonatal lupus, photosensitivity	Poor correlation
Arterial or venous thrombosis, pregnancy complications, thrombocytopenia	Complications of the antiphospholipid syndrome can occur even when "inflammatory" disease appears quiescent

- **Thrombocytopenia** – May be modest (platelet counts of 50,000–100,000/mm^3), chronic and asymptomatic, or profound (<20,000/mm^3) and acute, with gum bleeding, petechiae, and other complications. Thrombocytopenia in SLE has multiple potential causes, including immune thrombocytopenic purpura, the antiphospholipid syndrome, thrombotic thrombocytopenic purpura, and otherwise active SLE in which the mechanism of thrombocytopenia is not always clear.

Autoantibodies and Complement

- **ANA** – Positive ANA present in virtually all patients (high sensitivity), but present in many other conditions (low specificity). Typically in high titer and can present in any pattern; titer not useful in following course of disease.

- **dsDNA** – Antibodies to double-stranded DNA. High specificity for SLE. May be useful in predicting and assessing disease activity in selected patients, particularly those with renal disease.

- **Anti-Sm antibodies** – High diagnostic specificity. No unique associations with specific SLE manifestations. Titers do not track with disease activity.

- **SSA/Ro and SSB/La** – Occur in a subset of patients at increased risk of photosensitivity, dry eyes and dry mouth (secondary Sjögren's syndrome), subacute cutaneous lesions, and risk of having child with neonatal lupus.

- **Complement** – Low serum complement levels seen with active disease. Most commonly measured by C3, C4, or CH50 levels.

Diagnosis

- **Criteria** – American College of Rheumatology (ACR) has developed criteria for the classification of SLE. These criteria are not diagnostic criteria but rather are used for classifying patients for research studies. The presence of four or more criteria is required for classification of a patient as having SLE. Criteria are typically not present simultaneously but evolve over weeks, months, or even years.

Criteria for the Classification of Systemic Lupus Erythematosus[a]

Criterion	Definition
1. Malar rash	Fixed erythema, flat or raised, over malar eminences, tending to spare nasolabial folds
2. Discoid rash	Erythematous raised patches with adherent keratotic scaling and follicular plugging; atrophic scarring may occur in older lesions
3. Photosensitivity	Skin rash as a result of unusual reaction to sunlight, by patient history or physician observation
4. Oral ulcers	Oral or nasopharyngeal ulceration, usually painless, observed by physician
5. Arthritis	Nonerosive arthritis involving two or more peripheral joints, characterized by tenderness, swelling, or effusion
6. Serositis	a) Pleuritis – convincing history of pleuritic pain or rub heard by a physician or evidence of pleural effusion OR b) Pericarditis – documented by ECG or rub or evidence of pericardial effusion

Criterion	Definition
7. Renal disorder	a) Persistent proteinuria >0.5 g per day or >3+ if quantitation not performed *OR* b) Cellular casts – may be red cell, hemoglobin, granular, tubular, or mixed
8. Neurologic disorder	a) Seizures – in the absence of offending drugs or known metabolic derangements; e.g. uremia, ketacidosis, or electrolyte imbalance *OR* b) Psychosis – in the absence of offending drugs or known metabolic derangements; e.g. uremia, ketoacidosis, or electrolyte imbalance
9. Hematologic disorder	a) Hemolytic anemia – with reticulocytosis *OR* b) Leukopenia – <4,000/mm^3 total on two or more occasions *OR* c) Lymphopenia – <1,500/mm^3 on two or more occasions *OR* d) Thrombocytopenia – <100,000/mm^3 in the absence of offending drugs
10. Immunologic disorder[b]	a) Anti-DNA; antibody to native DNA in abnormal titer *OR* b) Anti-Sm; presence of antibody to the Sm nuclear antigen *OR* c) Positive finding of antiphospholipid antibodies based on (1) an abnormal serum level of IgG or IgM anti-cardiolipin antibodies; or (2) a positive test result for lupus anticoagulant using a strand method; or (3) a false-positive serologic test for syphilis known to b positive for at least 6 months and confirmed by a negative *Treponema pallidum* immobilization or fluorescent treponemal antibody absorption test
11. Antinuclear antibody	An abnormal titer of antinuclear antibody by immunofluorescence or an equivalent assay at any point in time and in the absence of drugs known to be associated with "drug-induced lupus" syndrome

[a] This classification is based on 11 criteria. For the purpose of identifying patients in clinical studies, a person must have SLE if any four or more of the 11 criteria are present, serially or simultaneously, during any interval of observation.

[b] The modifications to criterion number 10 were made in 1997.

Adapted from Tan EM, Cohen AS, Fries JF, et al. The 1982 revised criteria for the classification of systemic lupus erythematosus (SLE). Arthritis Rheum 1982; 25: 1271–1277. Copyright © 1982 American College of Rheumatology. Reproduced with permission of John Wiley & Sons, Inc.

Adapted from Hochberg MC. Updating the American College of Rheumatology revised criteria for the classification of systemic lupus erythematosus (letter). Arthritis Rheum 1997; 40: 1725. Copyright © 1997 American College of Rheumatology. Reproduced with permission of John Wiley & Sons, Inc.

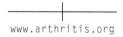

www.arthritis.org

- **Exclude RA** – Many features of SLE, including fatigue, symmetrical arthritis, serositis, and autoantibodies (antinuclear antibodies or rheumatoid factor), are similar to early signs and symptoms in rheumatoid arthritis. Distinguishing between these two diseases may be difficult.

Treatment

General Management

- **Patient education** – Crucial to optimizing clinical outcomes, as with any chronic illness.

- **Identify concomitant conditions** – Treat conditions that could contribute to fatigue, particularly hypothyroidism, anemia, fibromyalgia, and depression.

- **Photoprotection** – Patients who are photosensitive should be instructed to avoid excessive exposure to sunlight and routinely wear sunscreen and photoprotective clothing.

- **Review prescription drugs** – Some can exacerbate photosensitive reactions and other manifestations of systemic disease.

- **Infections** – Common in lupus; patients should be advised to seek medical attention urgently for unexplained fevers.

- **Pregnancies** – Considered high risk, because of potential disease flares in the mother and risk to the fetus. Anti-Ro/SSA and antiphospholipid antibodies are of particular concern.

- **Cardiovascular disease** – People with SLE are at increased risk for coronary artery disease. Attention to risk factors (e.g., hyperlipidemia, hypertension) and to primary and secondary prevention measures is important.

- **Osteoporosis** – Glucocorticoids and periods of inactivity because of active disease heighten the risk of poor bone health.

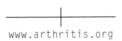

NSAIDs – Used widely for the treatment of musculoskeletal complaints, pleuritis, pericarditis, and headache.

● **Adverse effects of NSAIDs** – Effects on the kidneys, liver, and central nervous system that may be confused with worsening lupus activity.

Glucocorticoids – Effective in the management of many different manifestations of SLE.

● **Topical or intralesional preparations** – Often used for cutaneous lesions.

● **Intra-articular glucocorticoids** – Used occasionally for arthritis.

● **Oral or parenteral therapy** – Used for the control of systemic disease.

● **Low dose** – Oral administration, ranging from 5 mg to 30 mg prednisone daily, in single or divided doses, is effective in treating constitutional symptoms, cutaneous disease, arthritis, and serositis.

● **Higher dose** – More serious organ involvement, particularly nephritis, cerebritis, hematologic abnormalities, or systemic vasculitis, generally requires high-dose prednisone, 1–2 mg/kg/day.

Antimalarials – Some of the most commonly described medications for SLE. Include hydroxychloroquine, chloroquine, and quinacrine.

● **Uses** – Frequently used in the management of constitutional symptoms, cutaneous and musculoskeletal manifestations, and in some cases, serositis.

● **Combinations** – Synergy can be achieved in refractory cases of cutaneous disease with the combined use of either hydroxychloroquine or chloroquine with quinacrine.

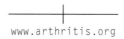

Azathioprine – Used as an alternative to cyclophosphamide for treatment of nephritis or as a steroid-sparing agent for nonrenal manifestations.

Mycophenolate mofetil – Now preferred to both cyclophosphamide and azathioprine for the management of moderate renal disease. Also used empirically for other SLE manifestations.

Recommended Monitoring Strategy for Drugs Commonly Used in Systemic Lupus Erythematosus

Drug	Toxicities requiring monitoring	Baseline evaluation
Salicylates, NSAIDs	Gastrointestinal bleeding, hepatic toxicity, renal toxicity, hypertension	CBC, creatinine, urinalysis, AST, ALT
Glucocorticoids	Hypertension, hyperglycemia, hyperlipidemia, hypokalemia, osteoporosis, osteonecrosis, cataract, weight gain, infections, fluid retention	BP, bone densitometry, glucose, potassium, cholesterol, triglycerides (HDL/LDL)
Hydroxychloroquine	Macular damage	None unless patient is over 40 years of age or has previous eye disease
Azathioprine	Myelosuppression, hepatotoxicity, lymphoproliferative disorders	CBC, platelet count, AST or ALT. Consider checking thiopurine methyltransferase level before starting azathioprine
Cyclophosphamide	Myelosuppression, myeloproliferative disorders, malignancy, immunosuppression, hemorrhagic cystitis, secondary infertility	CBC and differential and platelet count, urinalysis
Methotrexate	Myelosuppression, hepatic fibrosis, cirrhosis, pulmonary infiltrates, fibrosis	CBC, chest radiograph within past year, hepatitis B and C serology in high-risk patients, AST, albumin, bilirubin, creatinine

AST, aspartate transaminase; ALT, alanine transaminase; BP, blood pressure; CBC, complete blood cell count; HDL, high-density lipoprotein; LDL, low-density lipoprotein; Pap, Papanicolaou.

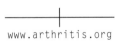

Cyclophosphamide – The mainstay of treatment for severe organ-system disease, particularly lupus nephritis.

Methotrexate – Continues to be used most commonly as a steroid-sparing agent for milder manifestations of disease. Particularly helpful in the arthritis of SLE.

Indicate review	Laboratory
Dark/black stool, dyspepsia, nausea/vomiting, abdominal pain, shortness of breath, edema	CBC and serum creatinine at each visit
Polyuria, polydipsia, edema, shortness of breath, BP at each visit, visual changes, bone pain	Urinary dipstick for glucose every visit, total cholesterol yearly, bone densitometry every other year
Visual changes	Fundoscopic and visual fields every 6–12 months
Symptoms of myelosuppression	CBC and platelet count every 1–2 weeks with changes in dose (every 1–3 months thereafter), AST yearly, Pap test at regular intervals
Symptoms of myleosuppression, hematuria, infertility	CBC and urinalysis monthly, urine cytology and Pap test yearly for life
Symptoms of myelosuppression, hematuria, infertility	CBC and urinalysis monthly, urine cytology and Pap test yearly for life

Reproduced from: Guidelines for referral and management of systemic lupus erythematosus in adults. American College of Rheumatology Ad Hoc Committee on Systemic Lupus Erythematosus. Arthritis Rheum 1999; 42: 1785–1796. Copyright © 1999 American College of Rheumatology. Reproduced with permission of John Wiley & Sons, Inc.

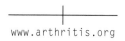

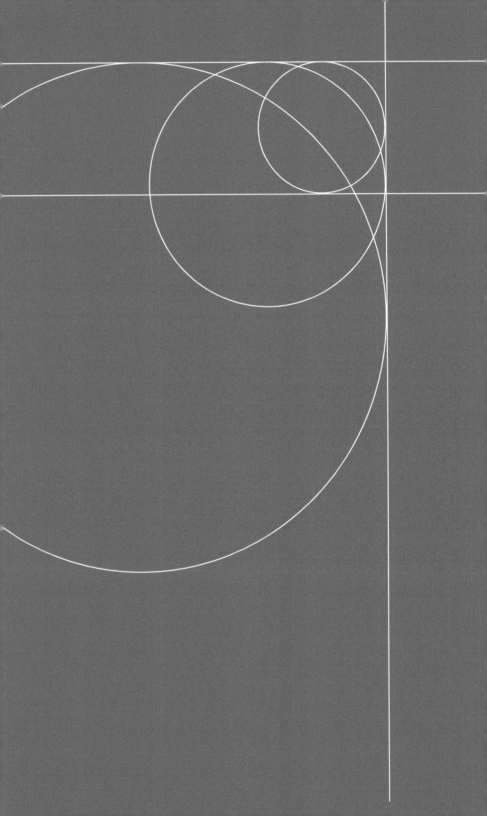

18 ANTIPHOSPHOLIPID SYNDROME

Antiphospholipid syndrome (APS) is an autoimmune disease associated with recurrent arterial or venous thromboses, pregnancy losses, livedo reticularis, and mild thrombocytopenia.

Clinical Features

- **Major clinical features** – Thrombosis and recurrent pregnancy losses.

- **Venous thromboses** – The deep veins of the leg are most frequently affected, but thrombosis also has been described in the pulmonary vessels, inferior vena cava, renal, hepatic (Budd–Chiari syndrome), axillary, and sagital veins.

- **Arterial thromboses** – Strokes or transient ischemic attacks are the most common presentations of arterial thrombosis, but myocardial, adrenal, and gastrointestinal infarction, and gangrene of the extremities may also occur.

- **Fetal death** – In the second or third trimester is characteristic of APS, but recurrent pregnancy loss can occur at any stage of gestation.

- **Other features** – Livedo reticularis, cardiac valvular vegetations (Libman–Sacks endocarditis), valvular insufficiency, pulmonary hypertension, leg ulcers, migraine headaches, and a variety of neurologic complications, including chorea, memory loss, dementia, multiple sclerosis-like syndromes, and transverse myelopathy.

Laboratory Features

- **Thrombocytopenia** – Mild-to-moderate thrombocytopenia (platelet counts in the range of 100,000–150,000/mm^3).

- **Anticardiolipin antibody** – Levels should be reported semi-quantitatively as high (>80 units), medium (20–80 units), or low (10–20 units). A medium-to-high positive IgG, IgM, or rarely, IgA anticardiolipin is most specific for the diagnosis of APS.

- **Lupus anticoagulant test** – Attributable to prolongation of clotting times by antiphospholipid antibodies in vitro.

Diagnosis

- **Criteria** – Classification criteria for APS are available.

Preliminary Classification Criteria for Antiphospholipid Syndrome

Vascular thrombosis
a) One or more clinical episodes of arterial, venous or small-vessel thrombosis in any tissue or organ *and*
b) Thrombosis confirmed by imaging or Doppler studies or histopathology, with the exception of superficial venous thrombosis *and*
c) For histopathologic confirmation, thrombosis present without significant evidence of inflammation in the vessel wall.

Pregnancy morbidity
a) One or more unexplained deaths of a morphologically normal fetus at or beyond the 10th week of gestation, with normal fetal morphology documented by ultrasound or by direct examination of the fetus *or*
b) One or more premature births of a morphologically normal neonate at or before the 34th week of gestation because of severe pre-eclampsia or severe placental insufficiency *or*
c) Three or more unexplained consecutive spontaneous abortions before the 10th week of gestation, with maternal anatomic and hormonal abnormalities and paternal and maternal chromosomal causes excluded.

Laboratory criteria
a) Anticardiolipin antibody of IgG and/or IgM isotype in blood, present in medium or high titer on two or more occasions at least six weeks apart, measured by standard enzyme-linked immunosorbent assay for beta-2-glycoprotein-1 dependent anticardiolipin antibodies *or*
b) Lupus anticoagulant present in plasma on two or more occasions at least six weeks apart, detected according to the guidelines of the International Society on Thrombosis and Hemostasis.

Definite APS is considered to be present if at least one of the clinical and one of the laboratory criteria are met.

Adapted from Wilson WA, Gharavi AE, Koike T, et al. International consensus statement on preliminary classification criteria for definite antiphospholipid syndrome. Report of an International Workshop. Arthritis Rheum 1999; 42: 1309–1311. Copyright © 1999 American College of Rheumatology. Reproduced with permission from John Wiley & Sons, Inc.

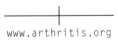

- **Consider APS** – In patients with unexplained arterial or venous thrombosis (particularly in people younger than 50 years), thrombosis at unusual sites (e.g. renal or adrenal veins), recurrent thrombotic events, or women with recurrent second- or third-trimester pregnancy losses.

- **Exclude** – Other diagnoses that should be considered in people with unexplained venous thrombosis include factor V Leiden (activated protein C resistance); protein C, protein S, or antithrombin III deficiency; dysfibrinogenemias; abnormalities of fibrinolysis; nephrotic syndrome; polycythemia vera; Behçet's syndrome; paroxysmal nocturnal hemoglobinuria; and thrombosis associated with oral contraceptives. In patients with arterial occlusions, the differential diagnosis includes hyperlipidemias, diabetes mellitus, hypertension, vasculitis, sickle cell disease, homocystinuria, and Buerger's disease.

Treatment

- **Oral anticoagulants** – Prophylaxis with warfarin indicated in people who have APS and recurrent venous or arterial thrombosis.

- **Subcutaneous heparin** – Pregnancy outcome can be markedly improved by using subcutaneous heparin at low doses of 5,000–10,000 units twice a day, plus one low-dose daily aspirin.

- **Intravenous gamma globulin** – If pregnancy loss occurs despite heparin, four-day or five-day pulses of intravenous gamma globulin (0.4 g/kg/day) given monthly, plus one low-dose daily aspirin, may be effective and safe.

- **Immunosuppressive therapy** – Has little or no role in the treatment of this syndrome.

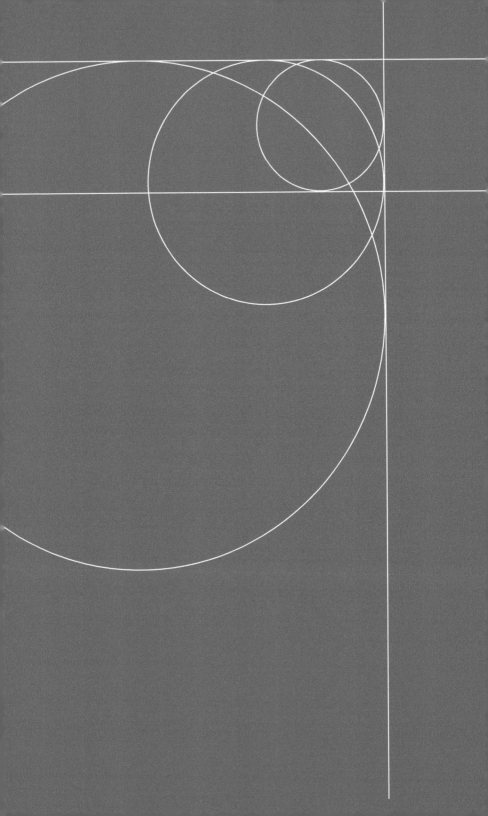

19 SYSTEMIC SCLEROSIS

Systemic sclerosis (SSc; scleroderma) is a chronic multisystem disease characterized by fibrosis of the skin and the internal organs including the lungs, kidneys, and gastrointestinal tract.

Clinical Features

- **Initial symptoms** – Typically are nonspecific and include Raynaud's phenomenon, fatigue or lack of energy, and musculoskeletal complaints.

- **Subsets** – Systemic sclerosis is classified into subsets of disease defined by the degree of clinically involved skin.

Raynaud's Phenomenon

- **Reversible vasospasm of digital vessels** – Occurs in more than 90% of people with SSc. Associated with color changes of the skin of the digits. Attacks triggered by cold temperature or emotional stress.

- **Tissue damage** – May be seen in patients with chronic or severe Raynaud's resulting in tissue fibrosis of the fingers (sclerodactyly), loss of tissue from the digital pads ("digital pitting"), digital ulceration, and on occasions, ischemic demarcation and the need for digital surgery or amputation.

Skin

- **Early changes** – In the earliest stage of disease, the skin appears mildly inflamed with nonpitting edema and, in some cases, erythema, and pruritus. Over time, collagen deposition leads to thickening of the dermis, with gradual damage to the normal skin and its appendages. The patient notices tightening of the skin and decreased flexibility.

- **Late changes** – As SSc progresses into the fibrotic stage, the skin becomes more thickened, and severe drying of the surface often leads to pruritus. The skin then becomes atrophic and thinned, with tethering secondary to the binding of fibrotic tissue to underlying structures.

Subsets of Systemic Sclerosis

Diffuse cutaneous systemic sclerosis
• Proximal skin thickening involving face/neck, trunk, and symmetrically, the fingers, hands, arms and legs • Rapid onset of disease following appearance of Raynaud's phenomenon • Significant visceral disease: lung, heart, gastrointestinal, or kidney • Associated with antinuclear antibodies and absence of anticentromere antibody • Variable disease course but overall poor prognosis: survival 40–60% at 10 years
Limited cutaneous systemic sclerosis
• Skin thickening limited to symmetrical change of fingers, distal arms, legs, and face/neck • Progression of disease after onset of Raynaud's phenomenon • Late visceral disease with prominent hypertension and digital amputation • CREST syndrome • Association with anticentromere antibody • Relatively good prognosis: survival ≥70% at 10 years
Overlap syndromes
• Diffuse or limited systemic sclerosis with typical features of one or more of the other connective-tissue diseases • Mixed connective-tissue disease: features of systemic lupus erythematosus, systemic sclerosis, polymyositis, rheumatoid arthritis, and presence of anti-U, RNP
Undefined connective-tissue disease
• Patients with features of systemic sclerosis who do not have definite clinical or laboratory findings to make a diagnosis
Localized scleroderma
• Morphea: plaques of fibrotic skin and subcutaneous tissue without systemic disease • Linear scleroderma: longitudinal fibrotic bands that occur predominantly on extremities and involve skin and deeper tissues

Musculoskeletal

● **Early features** – Musculoskeletal pain, arthritis, tendinitis, (often with tendon friction rubs), muscle weakness, and joint contractures are common, especially in people with diffuse cutaneous scleroderma.

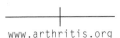

- **Nonspecific musculoskeletal complaints** – Arthralgias and myalgias are one of the earliest symptoms of SSc.

- **Pain and stiffness** – Generally are out of proportion to objective inflammatory signs.

- **Late features** – The dominant musculoskeletal problem in late SSc is muscle atrophy and weakness.

Pulmonary

- **Early features** – The most common initial symptom is dyspnea on exertion, without cough or chest pain.

- **Rales** – Velcro-like rales may be heard on chest auscultation, particularly in patients with pulmonary fibrosis.

- **Detection** – Periodic pulmonary function testing and 2D- echocardiography are the most effective methods of detection.

- **Course** – The majority of patients have early, but modest, declines in lung function tests and then follow stable courses reflecting inactive lung disease.

- **Mortality** – Lung failure is the leading cause of mortality in SSc.

Gastrointestinal

- **Mouth** – A small oral aperture, dry mucosal membranes, and periodontal disease (Sjögren's syndrome) can lead to problems with chewing foods, loss of teeth, and poor nutrition.

- **Upper esophagus** – Dysphagia and heartburn are the most common gastrointestinal symptoms found in SSc.

- **Lower esophagus** – Esophageal disease is associated with esophageal reflux, esophagitis, and delayed emptying of the stomach, leading to early satiety, bloating, nausea, and vomiting.

- **Small intestine** – Dysmotility of the small intestine may be asymptomatic, or it can cause severe distension, abdominal pain, and vomiting. Mild abdominal distension, crampy abdominal pain, diarrhea, weight loss, and malnutrition also can be consequences of malabsorption caused by bacterial overgrowth in stagnant intestinal fluids.

- **Large intestine** – As a consequence of muscular atrophy of the large bowel wall, asymptomatic wide-mouth diverticula unique to SSc commonly are found in the transverse and descending colon.

Cardiac

- **Clinical manifestations** – Often not seen until late in the course of the disease. Symptoms include dyspnea on exertion, palpitations, and less frequently, chest discomfort.

- **Pericardial effusion** – Can be demonstrated by echocardiography in 30–40% of primarily asymptomatic SSc patients.

Renal

- **Renal crisis** – Characterized by accelerated hypertension and/or rapidly progressive renal failure. Approximately 80% of cases of renal crisis occur within the first four or five years of disease, usually in patients with diffuse disease.

- **Outcome** – Poorer outcomes are more likely in men, patients with an older age of onset, and those who present with creatinine levels greater than 3 mg/dl.

- **Risk factors** – Renal crisis risk factors include diffuse skin disease, new unexplained anemia, use of glucocorticoids, pregnancy, and the presence of anti-RNA polymerase III antibodies.

Laboratory Features

- **Routine studies** – Routine chemistries and complete blood count should be obtained at baseline and at follow-up as necessary.

- **Antinuclear antibodies** – Positive in most patients, typically in a speckled pattern. Specific antinuclear antibodies (anticentromere, antitopoisomerase, and RNA polymerase, etc.) may be seen in subsets of SSc patients and help to predict the risk of future organ involvement and course.

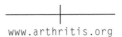

Diagnosis

- **Criteria** – The presence of one major or two minor criteria permits the diagnosis of systemic sclerosis.

Criteria for the Classification of Systemic Sclerosis (Scleroderma)

A. Major criterion
Proximal scleroderma: Symmetric thickening, tightening, and induration of the skin of the fingers and the skin proximal to the metacarpophalangeal or metatarsophalangeal joints. The changes may affect the entire extremity, face, neck, and trunk (thorax and abdomen).
B. Minor criteria
1. *Sclerodactyly:* Above-indicated skin changes limited to the fingers. 2. *Digital pitting scars or loss of substance from the finger pad:* Depressed areas at tips of fingers or loss of digital pad tissue as a result of ischemia. 3. *Bibasilar pulmonary fibrosis:* Bilateral reticular pattern of linear or lineonodular densities most pronounced in basilar portions of the lungs on standard chest roentgenogram; may assume appearance of diffuse mottling or "honeycomb lung." These changes should not be attributable to primary lung disease.

For the purposes of classifying patients in clinical trials, population surveys, and other studies, a person shall be said to have systemic sclerosis (scleroderma) if the one major or two or more minor criteria are present. Localized forms of scleroderma, eosinophilic fasciitis, and the various forms of pseudoscleroderma are excluded from these criteria.

Adapted from the Subcommittee for Scleroderma Criteria of the American Rheumatism Association Diagnostic and Therapeutic Criteria Committee. Preliminary criteria for the classification of systemic sclerosis (scleroderma). Arthritis Rheum 1980; 23: 581–590. Copyright © 1980 American College of Rheumatology. Reproduced with permission of John Wiley & Sons, Inc.

- **Capillary microscopy** – Enlarged capillary loops and loss of normal capillaries in the nailfold of the digits are physical signs that may help distinguish SSc from primary Raynaud's phenomenon.

Treatment

Raynaud's phenomenon

- **Prevent attacks** – All patients should be cautioned to avoid cold exposure when possible; to use layers of warm, loose-fitting clothing (including warm socks, headgear, and mittens/gloves) when in the cold; and to stop smoking.

- **Vasodilator therapy and oral analgesics** – Raynaud's that interferes with daily activities or is complicated by digital-tip ulcers may require vasodilator therapy and oral analgesics.

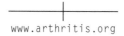

- **Necrosis** – Fingers and toes that are frankly necrotic or constantly blue/purple and painful require more aggressive treatment. Intravenous prostaglandin and prostacyclin may be infused. Medical lumbar or cervical sympathetic blocks may be used as primary treatment or as a way to determine the potential for reversal of vasospasm prior to performing permanent sympathectomies.

Skin

- **Topical moisturizers** – Because the skin's natural ability to moisturize is impaired in SSc, local skin care with topical moisturizers is essential.

- **Pruritus** – Can be very troublesome; oral antihistamines, topical analgesics, and topical glucocorticoids are worth trying.

- **Skin ulcers** – Should be kept clean with mild soap and water. Topical antibiotic ointments can be applied. Analgesics are important for pain control.

- **Subcutaneous calcinosis** – No treatment has been shown to treat or prevent subcutaneous calcinosis.

- **Colchicine** – A short course may reduce the inflammatory response to hydroxyapatite crystals.

Musculoskeletal

- **Goals** – Treatment should include measures to relieve pain, to stretch contractures, and to strengthen weak muscles.

- **Physical therapy** – Should be instituted early and aggressively in patients with rapidly progressive diffuse SSc and joint contractures.

- **Noninflammatory myopathy** – Myopathy with mildly elevated creatine kinase levels and deconditioning should be approached by muscle strengthening exercises.

- **NSAIDs** – May reduce pain and stiffness and improve joint function.

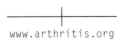

www.arthritis.org

- **Pure analgesics** – Also may be useful.

- **Glucocorticoids and methotrexate** – The drugs of choice for inflammatory myositis.

Gastrointestinal

- **Nonpharmacologic treatments** – Elevate the head of the bed, eat frequent small meals, avoid lying down within three or four hours of eating, and abstain from caffeine-containing beverages and cigarette smoking.

- **Pharmacologic therapies** – Oral antacids and H2 blockers may control minor reflux symptoms, but proton pump inhibitors (e.g., omeprazole and lansoprazole) are the drugs of choice for more severe complaints, such as esophageal strictures and recalcitrant reflux.

- **Promotility agents** – Gastroparesis frequently aggravates reflux and often underlies the symptoms of early satiety, nausea, and vomiting. Promotility agents (i.e., metoclopramide) may be helpful.

- **Broad-spectrum antibiotics** – Given in rotating, two-week courses may improve symptoms of small intestinal dysmotility.

- **Pseudo-obstruction** – Should be managed medically with nasogastric suction, bowel rest, and parenteral alimentation.

Kidneys

- **ACE inhibitors** – Reverse the hyperreninemia and hypertension characteristic of renal crisis.

- **Angiotensin-II receptor inhibitor** – Once renal crisis is controlled, the angiotensin-II receptor inhibitors may help maintain renal function and control hypertension.

- **Early detection** – Patients should take their blood pressure at home several times a week with goals of early introduction of ACE inhibitors and normalization of blood pressure.

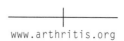

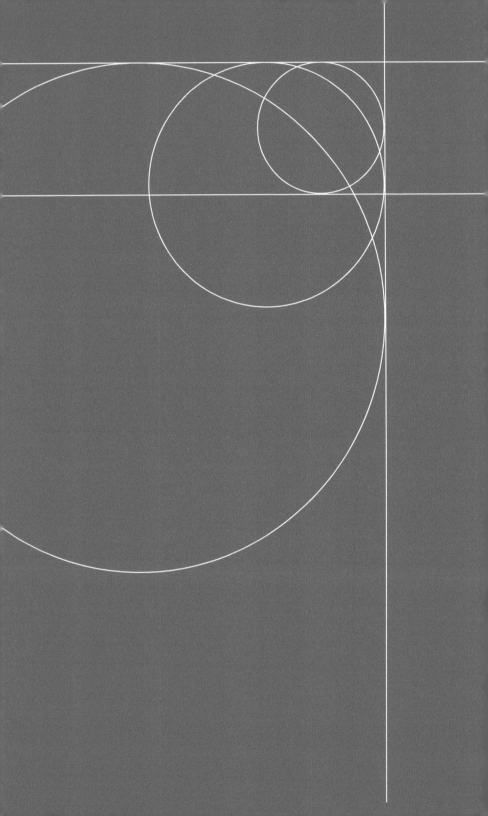

20 IDIOPATHIC INFLAMMATORY MYOPATHIES

The idiopathic inflammatory myopathies (IIMs) are a heterogeneous group of disorders characterized by symmetric proximal muscle weakness and elevated serum concentrations of enzymes derived from skeletal muscle.

Disease Subsets

The IIMs include several major distinct disease subsets:

- **Polymyositis** – Symmetric proximal muscle weakness and elevated serum concentrations of enzymes derived from skeletal muscle. Pelvic girdle and shoulder muscles are commonly affected.

- **Dermatomyositis** – Involves muscle groups similar to those affected by polymyositis but is associated with distinctive cutaneous features that may precede, develop simultaneously with, or follow symptoms of myopathy.

- **Juvenile dermatomyositis** – Dermatomyositis in children, which has multiple similarities to adult disease. Higher risk of muscle calcification and the development of systemic vasculitis.

- **Amyopathic dermatomyositis** – Cutaneous manifestations of dermatomyositis but with otherwise normal function and laboratory findings (good strength, normal enzymes, unremarkable electromyography and histology).

- **Inclusion body myositis (IBM)** – Occurs in the elderly and is characterized by a polymyositis-like presentation (although the specific muscles involved are more variable). Asymmetric distribution, distal weakness, or atrophy can occur alone or in combination with proximal weakness. Characteristic histopathology includes rimmed vacuoles.

Clinical Features

- **Onset** – Usual presentation is insidious, progressive, painless, symmetric, proximal muscle weakness. In contrast to the other IIMs, IBM is characterized frequently by distal, asymmetric involvement. The time course of onset is variable: several weeks; 3–6 months; and even 1–10 years.

- **Constitutional** – Fatigue, fever, and weight loss.

- **Other common manifestations** – Pitting edema of the extremities, periorbital regions, or eyelids, as well as hoarseness, dysphagia, nasal regurgitation of liquids, aspiration pneumonia, and dyspnea.

- **Malignancy** – Possible link between inflammatory myopathy and certain malignancies.

- **Extramuscular manifestations** – Lung involvement contributes significantly to the morbidity and mortality of myositis patients. Complications of rapidly progressive, diffuse alveolitis are particularly troublesome.

Laboratory Features

- **Elevated creatine kinase (CK)** – CK concentrations correlate well with disease activity in some but not all patients. Dermatomyositis, for example, is notorious for presenting with a low or normal CK concentration in the setting of profound muscle weakness.

- **Other serum muscle enzymes** – Aldolase, aspartate, and alanine aminotransferases (AST and ALT), and lactate dehydrogenase (LDH) are elevated in most cases.

- **Serum antibodies** – Antinuclear or anticytoplasmic antibodies are present in the majority of patients with IIM, with the exception of IBM. Some antibodies are termed myositis-specific autoantibodies (MSAs) because they are found exclusively in patients with features of an inflammatory myopathy. Examples of MSAs are the anti-synthetase antibodies (e.g. anti-Jo1), anti-Mi2 and anti-SRP antibodies.

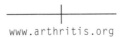

www.arthritis.org

Diagnosis

- **Muscle biopsy** – Gold standard in confirming a diagnosis of IIM. Different forms of IIM have distinctive histopathologic findings.

- **Skin biopsy** – In dermatomyositis, cutaneous histopathologic findings include vacuolar alteration of the epidermal basal layer, necrotic keratinocytes, vascular dilatation, and a perivascular lymphocytic infiltrate.

- **Electromyography (EMG)** – Allows for several muscle groups to be examined. The typical EMG features of myofibril irritability include fibrillation potentials, complex repetitive discharges, and positive sharp waves on needle insertion. In addition to aiding in the diagnosis, EMG is helpful in the selection of a site for muscle biopsy.

- **Magnetic resonance imaging (MRI)** – Can be used to document myositis or a disease flare, to distinguish chronic–active from chronic–inactive myositis, and to direct the site of biopsy.

- **High-resolution computed tomography (HRCT)** – In lung involvement, HRCT screening may reveal "ground glass" opacities (consistent with alveolitis), consolidation, subpleural lines or bands, traction bronchiectasis, and honeycombing (fibrosis).

- **Cinesophagogram** – Barium swallow used in myositis patients with proximal or distal dysphagia to demonstrate cricopharyngeal hypertrophy or spasm in the case of IBM; or poorly coordinated motion of the pharyngeal (striated) musculature, vallecular pooling, or aspiration of barium into the trachea in the case of severe polymyositis or dermatomyositis.

Treatment

- **Goal** – To preserve and improve existing muscle function, and prevent atrophy and muscle contractures.

- **Physical therapy** – Passive exercises and stretching in more severe cases of muscle weakness. Progressively more active sessions are possible as muscle strength improves.

- **Glucocorticoids** – Agents of choice for the initial treatment of IIM.

- **Methotrexate or azathioprine** – Effective in steroid-refractory patients and as steroid-sparing therapies.

- **Other immunosuppressive agents** – Cyclosporine and mycophenolate mofetil have shown some benefit. Immunosuppressive agents in IBM are generally not beneficial.

- **Intravenous immunoglobulin** – Appears to be particularly effective in some cases of dermatomyositis.

- **Biologic response modifiers** – Rituximab has demonstrated promise in case series.

- **Rash treatments** – Hydroxychloroquine, quinacrine, isotretinoin, topical tacrolimus, methotrexate, mycophenolate mofetil, or any of the other immunosuppressants can be used to treat the cutaneous lesions of dermatomyositis.

21 METABOLIC MYOPATHIES

The metabolic myopathies are a heterogeneous group of diseases characterized by impaired skeletal muscle energy production. They are divided into primary and secondary subtypes. Primary metabolic myopathies are associated with genetically determined defects in glycogen and lipid metabolism and in mitochondrial oxidative phosphorylation. These include the muscle glycogenoses and the lipid and mitochondrial myopathies. Secondary metabolic myopathies arise from endocrine or electrolyte abnormalities, and from therapy with specific drugs.

Diagnosis

- **Muscle symptoms** – The diagnosis of a metabolic myopathy should be suspected in a patient with muscle symptoms that develop during or after exercise, particularly if associated with myoglobinuria. Metabolic myopathies should also be included in the differential diagnosis of slowly progressive proximal or truncal muscle weakness.

- **Laboratory testing** – Support for the diagnosis of certain metabolic myopathies can be gained from the measurement of organic and amino acids in the blood and urine, and exercise testing (see Table).

- **Muscle biopsy and/or molecular genetic testing** – To confirm diagnosis.

Key Features of Primary Metabolic Myopathies

Biochemical class	Enzyme or biochemical defect	Genetics	Muscle symptoms
Defects in glycogenolysis or glycolysis (glycogenoses)	Myophosphorylase	AR	Exercise intolerance
	Phosphofructokinase	AR	Exercise intolerance, proximal myopathy (late onset)
	Phosphorylase b kinase	AR	Myopathy in childhood
		AR(?XR)	Exercise intolerance, myoglobinuria
	Phosphoglycerate mutase	AR	Exercise intolerance, myoglobinuria
	Lactate dehydrogenase	AR	Exercise intolerance, myoglobinuria
	Phosphoglycerate kinase	XR	Exercise intolerance, myoglobinuria
	Debrancher (adult patients)	AR	Generalized or distal weakness
	Brancher	AR	Progressive myopathy
	Aldolase	AR	Exercise intolerance, weakness
	Acid maltase (nonclassical forms)	AR	Progressive myopathy
Defects in fatty acid transport	Carnitine deficiency (primary systemic)	AR	Facial and proximal myopathy
	Carnitine deficiency (primary myopathic)	AR	Progressive myopathy
	Carnitine palmitoyltransferase II	AR	Exercise intolerance, myoglobinuria

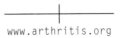

Other clinical features	Laboratory features	Diagnostic testing
Second-wind phenomenon	Variable ↑ serum CK	Abnormal FIET
Out-of-wind phenomenon, hemolytic anemia, gout	↑ serum CK, uric acid	Abnormal FIET
Hepatomegaly, fasting hypoglycemia	↑ serum CK	
	↑ serum CK	
Most often in African–Americans	↑ serum CK	Abnormal FIET
	LDH does not rise in proportion to serum CK	Abnormal FIET with elevated pyruvate/lactate ratio
Hemolytic anemia, CNS dysfunction	Variable ↑ serum CK	Abnormal FIET
Hepatomegaly, left or biventricular hypertrophy		
Cardiomyopathy, hepatomegaly		
Hemolytic anemia		
Respiratory insufficiency	Deficient alpha-glucosidase in leukocytes and muscle	Myotonic discharges on EMG
Hypoketotic hypoglycemia, encephalopathy, cardiomyopathy	Total serum carnitine <5% normal	Reduced muscle carnitine
	Normal serum carnitine levels, variable ↑ serum CK	Muscle carnitine levels <25% normal
	Serum CK normal between attacks	

Biochemical class	Enzyme or biochemical defect	Genetics	Muscle symptoms
Defects in fatty acid beta-oxidation	Multiple acyl coA dehydrogenase		Progressive myopathy
	Very-long-chain acyl coA dehydrogenase (adult phenotype)		Exercise intolerance, myoglobinuria
	Trifunctional protein enzyme		Myoglobinuria
Defects in respiratory chain function (mitochondrial myopathy)	Mutations in mtDNA or nDNA genes that determine mitochondrial respiratory chain function	Maternal Mendelian Sporadic	Exercise intolerance, ptosis, external ophthalmoplegia
Defects in purine nucleotide cycle	Myoadenylate deaminase	AR	

AR, autosomal recessive; CK, creatine kinase; DCA, dicarboxylic acid; EMG, electromyography; FIET, forearm ischemic exercise test; mtDNA, mitochondrial DNA; nDNA, nuclear DNA; XR, X-linked recessive.

Data from Vladutiu GD. Neurol Clin 2000; 18: 53–104; DiMauro S, Lamperti C. Muscle Nerve 2001; 24: 984–999; Cwik VA. Neurol Clin 2000; 18: 167–184; Olpin SE. Clin Lab 2005; 51: 289–306; DiMauro S, Schon EA. N Engl J Med 2003; 348: 2656–2668; Nardin RA, Johns DR. Muscle Nerve 2001; 24: 170–191.

Treatment

Muscle glycogenosis

- **Modified exercise regimens** – Recommended.

- **Modified diet** – A high-protein, low-carbohydrate diet is generally recommended for patients with myophosphorylase deficiency. Ingestion of sucrose before exercise can markedly improve exercise tolerance. Vitamin B6 and creatine supplementation may also be beneficial. Patients with phosphofructokinase deficiency should avoid high-carbohydrate diets.

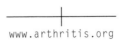

Other clinical features	Laboratory features	Diagnostic testing
	Increased urinary glutaric acid, increased plasma acyl-carnitine	
Peripheral neuropathy	Increased urinary DCAs	
Axonal neuropathy, ataxia, seizures, pigmentary retinopathy, sensorineural hearing loss	Elevation of resting, fasting blood lactate	Abnormal cycle ergometry
	None	Abnormal FIET

Secondary Metabolic Myopathies

- **Comorbidity** – Proximal muscle weakness is the primary feature of the myopathies that may accompany Cushing's syndrome, hypothyroidism, hyperthyroidism, vitamin D deficiency, acromegaly, and hyperparathyroidism. Hypothyroidism may be associated with elevation of serum creatine kinase and be misdiagnosed as an idiopathic inflammatory myopathy. Disorders that cause abnormally high or low concentrations of sodium, potassium, calcium, magnesium, or phosphorus can also cause weakness, fatigue, myalgias, or cramps.

- **Drugs** – Zidovudine may induce a mitochondrial myopathy.

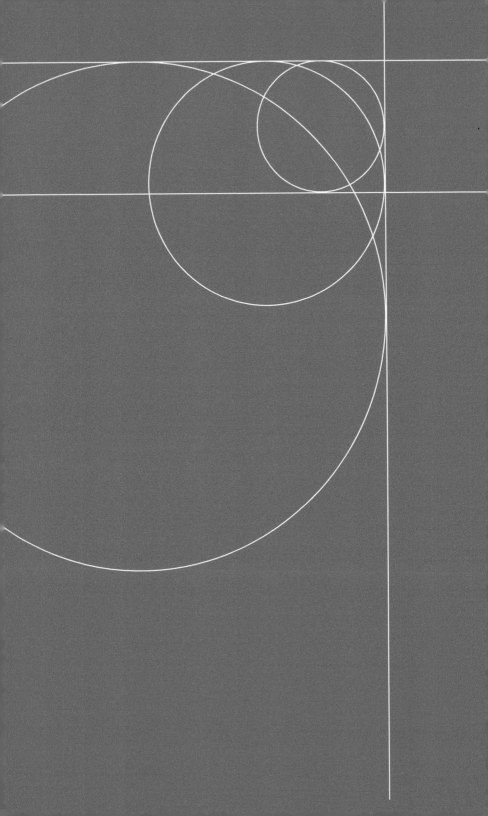

22 SJÖGREN'S SYNDROME

Sjögren's syndrome is an autoimmune disorder affecting exocrine glands. Dryness of the eyes and mouth are the two most common symptoms.

Clinical Features

- **Cardinal manifestations** – Oral and ocular symptoms and signs of dryness and the presence of autoantibodies.

- **Constitutional features** – Fatigue, myalgias, arthralgias, low-grade fever, and lymphadenopathy common.

Ocular Manifestations

- **Gritty eyes** – Sensation of sand or grit in the eyes often reported.

- **Matter** – Often present in morning at corners of eyes.

Oral Manifestations

- **Common oral symptoms** – Sensation of decreased saliva, oral dryness when eating, the need to drink liquids when swallowing dry foods, intolerance of spicy foods, altered taste, and a chronic burning sensation.

- **Oral examination** – Peridontal disease common and may lead to tooth erosions and caries, especially at the gingival margins and on the incisal edges of the teeth. Soft-tissue changes are particularly common on the tongue, which may become furrowed, and the mucosa may become dry and sticky.

- **Salivary glands** – Visible enlargement of the major salivary glands.

Cutaneous

- **Dry skin** – Often associated with pruritus and decreased sweating.

Thyroid

- **Thyroid disease** – Particularly hypothyroidism, is common.

Respiratory

- **Nonproductive cough** – Common and due to tracheal dryness and a diminution in mucus production.

- **Progressive pulmonary disease** – Unusual.

Musculoskeletal

- **Symmetrical polyarthritis** – Resembles rheumatoid arthritis, but is nondeforming and tends to respond well to standard treatments used in rheumatoid arthritis.

Neurologic

- **Peripheral neuropathy** – A variety of forms of neuropathy can occur in Sjögren's syndrome, ranging from mononeuritis multiplex to small fiber sensory neuropathy to dorsal root gangliopathy and others. The most common type of peripheral neuropathy in Sjögren's syndrome has a predilection for the lower extremities, leading to numbness, tingling, and burning.

Hematologic

- **Lymphoid malignancy** – There is a 44-fold increase in the frequency of B-cell lymphomas among people with Sjögren's syndrome.

Reproductive

- **Vaginal dryness** – Associated with dyspareunia.

Urinary Tract

- **Irritable bladder** – Symptoms not uncommon.

- **Increased urinary frequency** – May relate to increased fluid intake to alleviate oral dryness.

- **Renal abnormalities** – Diminished ability to concentrate urine occurs in about half of all cases.

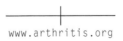

Laboratory Features

- **Autoantibodies** – Anti-Ro/SSA, anti-La/SSB, and rheumatoid factor (RF) are hallmarks of Sjögren's syndrome. Hypergammaglobulinemia is common in Sjögren's syndrome, and a majority of cases are associated with the presence of RF (90%), or anti-Ro/SSA or anti-La/SSB (50–90%).

- **Antinuclear antibodies** – Present in about 80% of cases.

Tests

- **Minor salivary gland biopsy** – Focal mononuclear cell infiltrates of exocrine tissues are hallmarks of Sjögren's syndrome, and best documented with salivary gland biopsy.

- **Schirmer's test** – Strip of filter paper placed over bottom eyelid to measure tear formation. Five mm or less of wetting in five minutes is abnormal.

- **Fluorescein tear film** – Break-up time of less than 10 seconds (observed on slit lamp examination) suggests dry eyes.

- **Staining** – Rose Bengal dye staining may be used to detect damage to ocular surface.

Diagnosis

- **Criteria** – The American-European Consensus Group has developed revised criteria.

Revised International Classification Criteria for Sjögren's Syndrome

I. Ocular symptoms: a positive response to at least one of the following questions:
   a. Have you had daily, persistent, troublesome dry eyes for more than three months?
   b. Do you have a recurrent sensation of sand or gravel in the eyes?
   c. Do you use tear substitutes more than three times a day?

II. Oral symptoms: a positive response to at least one of the following questions:
   a. Have you had a daily feeling of dry mouth for more than three months?
   b. Have you had recurrently or persistently swollen salivary glands as an adult?
   c. Do you frequently drink liquids to aid in swallowing dry food?

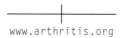

III. Ocular signs: objective evidence of ocular involvement defined as a positive result for at least one of the following tests:
  a. Schirmer's test, performed without anesthesia (≤5 mm in 5 minutes).
  b. Rose Bengal score or other ocular dry score (≥4 according to van Bijsterveld's scoring system).

IV. Histopathology of minor salivary glands: obtained through normal-appearing mucosal focal lymphocytic sialoadenitis, evaluated by an expert histopathologist, focal score ≥1, defined as a number of lymphocytic foci adjacent to normal-appearing mucous acini and containing more than 50 lymphocytes per 4 mm² of glandular tissue.

V. Salivary gland involvement: objective evidence of salivary gland involvement defined by a positive result for at least one of the following diagnostic tests:
  a. Unstimulated whole salivary flow (≤1.5 ml in 15 minutes).
  b. Parotid sialography showing the presence of diffuse sialectasias (punctuate, cavitary or destructive pattern), without evidence of obstruction in the major ducts.
  c. Salivary scintigraphy showing delayed uptake, reduced concentration and/or delayed excretion of tracer.

VI. Autoantibodies: presence in the serum of the following autoantibodies: Antibodies to SSA/Ro or SSB/La antigens, or both.

Revised Rules for Classification of Sjögren's Syndrome

For primary Sjögren's syndrome

In patients without any potentially associated disease, primary Sjögren's syndrome may be defined as follows:

a. The presence of any four of the six items is indicative of primary Sjögren's syndrome, as long as either item IV (Histopathology) or VI (Serology) is positive.

b. The presence of any three of the four objective criteria items (i.e. items III, IV, V, VI).

c. The classification tree procedure represents a valid alternative method for classification, although it should be more properly used in clinical-epidemiological surveys.

For secondary Sjögren's syndrome

In patients with a potentially associated disease (for example, another well-defined connective-tissue disease), the presence of item I or item II plus any two from among items III, IV, and V may be considered as indicative of secondary Sjögren's syndrome.

Exclusion criteria

Past history of head and neck radiation therapy, hepatitis C infection, acquired immunodeficiency disease (AIDS), pre-existing lymphoma, sarcoidosis, graft-versus-host disease, use of anticholinergic drugs (within four half-lives of the drug).

- **Exclusions** – Listed in criteria table.

- **Exclude other causes of dry eyes** – Other lacrimal gland diseases, lacrimal duct obstruction, loss of reflex tearing, and contact lenses.

- **Exclude other causes of dry mouth** – Many medications can cause dry mouth symptoms, including drugs commonly prescribed for hypertension, depression, and insomnia. Radiation therapy for head and neck tumors may result in profound symptoms or oral dryness.

Treatment

- **Self-management** – Help patients develop strategies for self-management and coping with physical, mental, and social challenges associated with their condition.

- **Artificial tears** – Instilled as drops into the eyes frequently to ameliorate symptoms.

- **Eye ointments** – Typically are used only at night, since they are viscous and may interfere with vision.

- **Topical glucocorticoids, cyclosporine, and intraocular androgens** – Growing evidence to suggest these may be beneficial for keratoconjunctivitis sicca.

- **Systemic pilocarpine** – Approved for the treatment of dry mouth, probably also improves ocular symptoms.

- **Punctal plugs** – May be inserted in refractory cases.

- **Dental care** – Frequent care important.

- **Caries prevention** – Daily topical fluoride used and antimicrobial mouth rinse.

- **Replace medications** – Medications that promote oral dryness or its complications should be replaced.

- **Artificial saliva and lubricants** – May ameliorate symptoms.

- **Sugar-free chewing gum or candies** – May stimulate salivary secretions.

- **Secretagogues** – May increase secretions in patients with sufficient exocrine tissue.

- **Hydroxychloroquine** – For milder systemic manifestations of autoimmune disorders, such as fever, rashes, and arthritis.

- **Immunomodulatory drugs** – Methotrexate, prednisone, azathioprine used in patients with prominent systemic manifestations.

23 VASCULITIDES

Giant Cell Arteritis, Polymyalgia Rheumatica, and Takayasu's Arteritis

Giant cell arteritis (GCA) and Takayasu's arteritis (TA) are two major forms of large-vessel vasculitis. They tend to involve the aorta, its primary branches, and (particularly in the case of GCA) medium-sized arteries of the head and neck. Polymyalgia rheumatica (PMR) can accompany, precede, or follow GCA, but it also occurs independently.

Clinical Features

GCA

- **Onset** – Aged ≥50 years.

- **Cranial GCA** – Headaches, scalp tenderness, ischemic neuropathy, jaw claudication, PMR, and occasionally posterior circulation events in the central nervous system (CNS).

- **Generalized inflammatory syndrome** – Fever and occasionally chills, night sweats, anorexia, and weight loss.

- **Large vessel GCA/aortitis** – Aortic arch syndrome – claudication of the arms, absent or asymmetrical pulses, and paresthesias. Aortic aneurysm or aortic insufficiency can develop years after diagnosis.

Isolated PMR

- **Muscle pain/stiffness** – Typically, myalgias are symmetrical and initially affect the shoulders. Also affect the neck, lower back, hips, and thighs.

- **Constitutional features** – Anorexia, weight loss, malaise, and depression.

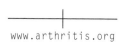

TA

- **Onset** – Adolescent girls and young women.

- **Generalized inflammatory syndrome** – Fever and chills, anorexia and weight loss, night sweats, malaise, and diffuse myalgias can predominate in early phases.

- **Carotid and vertebral artery involvement** – Neurologic and ophthalmologic symptoms.

- **Claudication** – Jaw and arm claudication caused by occlusion of the carotid and subclavian arteries, respectively.

- **Pulselessness** – Through involvement of the subclavian artery. Tends to affect upper extremities rather than lower ("reverse coarctation"), but legs can also be affected.

- **Cardiac disease** – Related to aortitis of the ascending aorta or severe hypertension.

- **Aortic regurgitation** – Usually results from dilatation of the ascending aorta, but occasionally valvular inflammation also present.

- **Myocardial ischemia** – Coronary arteries can be involved directly or indirectly.

- **Aneurysms** – Progressively enlarging aneurysms and possible rupture are a major concern in patients with TA of the aortic arch and the descending thoracic aorta.

- **Gastrointestinal (GI) symptoms** – Nausea, vomiting, and ischemic bowel disease.

Laboratory Features

GCA

- **Acute-phase reactants** – Highly elevated erythrocyte sedimentation rate (ESR) and C-reactive protein (CRP).

- **Anemia** – Mild-to-moderate normochromic or hypochromic anemia.

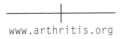

- **Platelets** – Thrombocytosis is common.

- **Liver function tests** – Alkaline phosphatase elevation is the classic abnormality, though it occurs in only a minority of patients.

Diagnosis

- **Vaso-occlusive disease and systemic inflammation** – GCA should be suspected if aged ≥50 years; TA in younger patients; PMR if prompt response to glucocorticoids.

- **Temporal artery biopsy** – Essential whenever possible for the diagnosis of GCA.

- **Bruits** – The detection of bruits over arteries can be helpful in making the diagnosis. Most common sites of detection are the subclavian, carotid, and femoral arteries.

- **Aortography** – Useful for direct measurement of the central aortic pressure, which is essential if occlusive disease is present in all four extremities.

- **Differential diagnosis for PMR** – Lack of the classic PMR response to moderate doses of glucocorticoids (prednisone 15–20 mg/day) suggests that the diagnosis of PMR should be reconsidered.

Treatment

- **Glucocorticoids** – Highly effective in suppressing clinical manifestations in GCA, TA, and isolated PMR.

- **Aspirin** – Doses ranging from 81 mg/day to 325 mg/day may be beneficial for reducing the risk of visual loss and CNS ischemic events in GCA.

- **Methotrexate** – Data on its potential for steroid sparing are mixed.

Polyarteritis Nodosa

- Polyarteritis nodosa (PAN) affects medium-sized, muscular arteries.

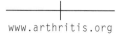

www.arthritis.org

Clinical Features

- **Fibrinoid necrosis** – Within the walls of affected blood vessels (arteries, not veins).

- **Microaneurysms** – An angiographic hallmark of PAN; also evident in the rare cases of PAN that come to autopsy.

- **Constitutional symptoms** – Fever, fatigue, malaise, myalgias, and arthralgias.

- **Kidneys** – Most commonly involved organ. Renin-mediated hypertension and renal insufficiency may result.

- **Cutaneous manifestations** – Livedo reticularis (racemosa), nodules, ulcerations, and frank ischemia of digits. Cutaneous PAN is a variant ostensibly limited to the skin.

- **Neuropathy** – Involvement of the peripheral nervous system is seen in 50–75% of patients, usually as an asymmetric sensory and motor neuropathy due to ischemia of peripheral nerves. Infarction of nerves results in mononeuritis multiplex.

- **GI symptoms** – Occur in 50% of patients. Post-prandial periumbilical pain or intestinal angina, nausea, vomiting, diarrhea, and GI bleeding.

- **Testicular pain or tenderness** – Occurs in ~33% of patients.

- **Coronary involvement** – Detected only at autopsy.

Laboratory Features

- **Antineutrophil cytoplasmic antibodies (ANCA)** – Patients with PAN do not have ANCA directed against either proteinase-3 (PR3) or myeloperoxidase (MPO) in their sera. The fact that PAN is a "seronegative" disease, not associated with a known autoantibody, often contributes to the difficulty in making this diagnosis.

Diagnosis

- **Physical examination** – Cutaneous features (livedo, nodules, ulcers, digital ischemia) and signs of vasculitic neuropathy (muscle wasting, foot- or wrist-drop) often evident.

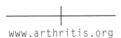

- **Angiography** – Guided by symptoms; abnormal arteriograms often reveal characteristic strictures or aneurysms.

- **Biopsy** – Guided by symptoms; skin, muscle, and peripheral nerve biopsies to aid diagnosis.

- **Differential diagnosis** – Criteria have been developed by the American College of Rheumatology (ACR) to help distinguish PAN from other vasculitides and rheumatic disorders.

ACR Classification of PAN

At least three of 10 criteria:
1. Weight loss ≥4 kg
2. Livedo reticularis
3. Testicular pain or tenderness
4. Myalgias, weakness, or leg tenderness
5. Mononeuropathy or polyneuropathy
6. Diastolic blood pressure >90 mm Hg
7. Elevated serum nitrogen urea (>40 mg/dl) or creatinine (>1.5 mg/dl)
8. Hepatitis B virus infection
9. Arteriographic abnormality
10. Biopsy of small- or medium-sized artery containing polymorphonuclear neutrophils

From: Lightfoot RW, et al. Arthritis Rheum 1990; 33: 1088–1093. Copyright © 1990 American College of Rheumatology. Reproduced with permission of John Wiley & Sons, Inc.

Treatment

- **Glucocorticoids** – About half of cases will be cured with glucocorticoids alone.

- **Cyclophosphamide** – In cases of rapidly progressive, or life- or organ-threatening PAN, cyclophosphamide should be added to glucocorticoid treatment.

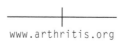

The Antineutrophil Cytoplasmic Antibody-Associated Vasculitides: Wegener's Granulomatosis, Microscopic Polyangiitis and the Churg–Strauss Syndrome

Wegener's granulomatosis (WG), microscopic polyangiitis (MPA), and the Churg–Strauss syndrome (CSS) are often grouped together under the term ANCA-associated vasculitides (AAVs). Most patients, particularly those with WG or MPA, have ANCA in their serum.

Key Clinical features of ANCA-associated Vasculitides

Feature	Wegener's granulomatosis
ANCA positivity	80–90%
ANCA antigen specificity	PR3 > MPO
Fundamental histology	Leukocytoclastic vasculitis; necrotizing, granulomatous inflammation (rarely seen in renal biopsy specimens)
Ear/nose/throat	Nasal septal perforation; saddle-nose deformity; conductive or sensorineural hearing loss; subglottic stenosis
Eye	Orbital pseudotumor; scleritis (risk of scleromalacia perforans); episcleritis; uveitis
Lung	Nodules, infiltrates, or cavitary lesions; large airway disease leading to bronchial narrowing; alveolar hemorrhage
Kidney	Segmental necrotizing glomerulonephritis; rare granulomatous features
Heart	Occasional valvular lesions
Peripheral nerve	Vasculitic neuropathy (10%)
Eosinophilia	Occasional and mild

ANCAs, antineutrophil cytoplasmic antibodies; MPO, myeloperoxidase; PR3, proteinase 3.
Reprinted from the American Journal of Medicine. Volume 117, Seo P, Stone JH.
The antineutrophil cytoplasmic antibody-associated vasculitides. pp 39–50.
Copyright © 2004, with permission from Elsevier.

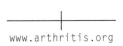

Clinical Features

- **Skin** – Palpable purpura, vesiculobullous lesions, papules, ulcers, digital infarctions, and splinter hemorrhages can all occur in AAVs. In both CSS and WG, cutaneous nodules known as Churg–Strauss granulomas may occur at sites that are also common locations for rheumatoid nodules.

- **Arthritis/arthralgias** – Joint problems are frequently the present-ing complaint. Migratory oligoarthritis is common.

- **GI involvement** – Less common in WG than in CSS and MPA.

Microscopic polyangiitis	Churg–Strauss syndrome
70%	50%
MPO > PR3	MPO > PR3
Leukocytoclastic vasculitis; no granulomatous inflammation	Eosinophilic tissue infiltrates and vasculitis; granulomas show eosinophilic necrosis
Absent or mild	Nasal polyps; allergic rhinitis; conductive hearing loss
Occasional eye disease: scleritis, episcleritis, uveitis	Occasional eye disease: scleritis, episcleritis, uveitis
Alveolar hemorrhage	Asthma; fleeting infiltrates; alveolar hemorrhage
Segmental necrotizing glomerulonephritis	Segmental necrotizing glomerulonephritis
Rare	Heart failure
Vasculitic neuropathy (58%)	Vasculitic neuropathy (78%)
None	All patients

Diagnosis

- **Histopathology** – Gold standard for diagnosis in most cases.

- **Exclude rheumatoid arthritis (RA)** – The combination of joint complaints, cutaneous nodules, and the high frequency of rheumatoid factor positivity among patients with AAV often leads to the misdiagnosis of RA early in the disease course.

Differential Diagnosis of ANCA-associated Vasculitides

Exclude	Specific disorders
Another form of AAV	WG, CSS, MPA, drug-induced AAV, or renal-limited vasculitis
Another form of vasculitis; typical vasculitic mimickers	Polyarteritis nodosa, Henoch–Schönlein purpura, cryoglobulinemia, antiglomerular basement membrane disease
Systemic inflammatory disorders associated with autoimmunity	Systemic lupus erythematosus, sarcoidosis, inflammatory bowel disease, relapsing polychondritis
Infection	Endocarditis, sepsis, deep fungal infections, mycobacteria (*Mycobacterium tuberculosis* and *Mycobacterium avium-intracellulare*), actinomycosis, syphilis
Malignancy	Lymphomatoid granulomatosis, lymphoma, Castleman's disease, lung tumors
Hypereosinophilic disorders	Allergic bronchopulmonary aspergillosis, chronic eosinophilic pneumonia, eosinophilic gastroenteritis, eosinophilic fasciitis, hypereosinophil syndrome, eosinophilic leukemia
Miscellaneous	Idiopathic pulmonary alveolar hemorrhage, cocaine-induced midline destructive lesions

AAV, ANCA-associated vasculitis; ANCA, antineutrophil cytoplasmic antibodies; CSS, Churg–Strauss syndrome; MPA, microscopic polyangiitis; WG, Wegener's granulomatosis.

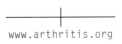

Treatment

Glucocorticoids are the cornerstone of therapy in the AAVs. WG and MPA nearly always require an additional agent (rituximab, cyclophosphamide, methotrexate) to control the disease.

- **Rituximab** – The preferred agent for remission induction in patients with severe WG or MPA. Role in CSS not clear.

- **Cyclophosphamide** – Now the second-line agent for the treatment of severe disease, because of toxicity concerns.

- **Azathioprine or methotrexate** – For remission–maintenance therapy. Methotrexate may be used to induce remission in cases of limited WG.

- **Glucocorticoids** – Some cases of CSS can be treated with monotherapy. Low doses of prednisone can be used to control recurrent disease flares.

Immune Complex-Mediated Vasculitides

The immune complex-mediated vasculitides are a clinically heterogeneous group of disorders linked by inefficient, defective, or dysregulated clearance of immune complexes by the reticuloendothelial system. There are four principal subtypes: hypersensitivity vasculitis; cryoglobulinemic vasculitis; Henoch–Schönlein purpura (HSP); and hypocomplementemic urticarial vasculitis.

Clinical Features

Hypersensitivity Vasculitis (sometimes termed "cutaneous leukocytoclastic angiitis")

- **ACR criteria** – At least three of the following: aged >16 years; use of a possible offending medication in temporal relation to the symptoms; palpable purpura; maculopapular rash; and biopsy of a skin lesion showing neutrophils around an arteriole or venule.

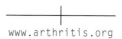

Cryoglobulinemic Vasculitis

- **Neurologic manifestations** – Dizziness, confusion, headache, and stroke caused by hyperviscosity syndrome in type I cryoglobulinemia.

- **Vascular stasis** – Type I can also be associated with livedo reticularis, acrocyanosis, and digital gangrene.

- **Purpura, arthralgias, and myalgias** – Triad of manifestations common in types II and III.

- **Systemic** – Includes membranoproliferative glomerulonephritis, peripheral neuropathy, and cutaneous ulcerations. More common in type II than in type III cryoglobulinemia.

HSP

- **IgA deposition** – Associated with leukocytoclastic vasculitis and intense IgA deposition within the walls of involved blood vessels.

- **Antecedent infection** – Many cases occur after upper respiratory tract infections. Group A streptococci, mycoplasma, Epstein–Barr virus, and varicella have all been implicated. HSP can also be induced by medications, e.g., antibiotics.

- **ACR criteria** – At least two of the following: aged ≤20 years; palpable purpura; bowel angina; and granulocytes in arteriole or venule walls on biopsy.

Hypocomplementemic Urticarial Vasculitis

- **Urticaria** – Purpuric lesions, often associated with moderate pain, burning, and tenderness with pruritus, last for days, and often worsen without therapy.

- **Arthralgias and myalgias** – Common in urticarial vasculitis.

- **Hypocomplementemic urticarial vasculitis syndrome (HUVS)** – Consists of the constellation of low complement levels and urticaria for a period of at least 6 months, as well as some or all of the following: arthritis, glomerulonephritis, scleritis, uveitis, angioedema, chronic obstructive pulmonary disease, pleurisy, and pericarditis.

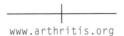

Diagnosis

- **Biopsy** – Diagnostic method of choice.

- **Light microscopy** – To demonstrate presence of leukocytoclastic vasculitis.

- **Direct immunofluorescence** – Can be diagnostic in immune complex-mediated vasculitis by illustrating the particular type and pattern of immunoreactants. In HSP, for example, direct immunofluorescence reveals florid immunoglobulin A deposition.

- **Serological testing** – Where biopsy is not feasible in patients with cryoglobulinemic vasculitis. The most relevant test is a serum cryoglobulin test. However, only a minority of patients with detectable cryoglobulins in their serum develop cryoglobulinemic vasculitis.

- **Exclude systemic lupus erythematosus** – Interface dermatitis as well as immunoreactant deposition within blood vessels are diagnostic of hypocomplementemic urticarial vasculitis. HUVS, in contrast, is a clinical diagnosis based not only on the presence of urticarial vasculitis but also on the occurrence of typical features in extracutaneous organ systems.

Treatment

- **Underlying cause** – Removal of inciting agent in hypersensitivity vasculitis. Treatment of the underlying cause of the cryoglobulins in cryoglobulinemic vasculitis (usually hepatitis C virus infection, sometimes Sjögren's syndrome, or another connective-tissue disease).

- **Glucocorticoids** – Help some disease manifestations in all patients, but not all. Generally effective in other forms of immune complex-mediated vasculitis.

- **Immunosuppressants** – Few data related to the use of cyclophosphamide, azathioprine, and other agents, but empiric use not uncommon in severe cases.

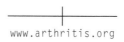

- **Biologic agents** – Rituximab can be useful in cryoglobulinemic vasculitis. Anecdotal data support trials of tumor necrosis factor inhibition in hypocomplementemic urticarial vasculitis, particularly for refractory disease manifestations (e.g., scleritis).

Miscellaneous Vasculitis (Primary Angiitis of the Central Nervous System, Cogan's Syndrome, and Erythema Elevatum Diutinum)

Clinical Features

Primary Angiitis of the Central Nervous System (PACNS)

- **Headache** – Most common symptom with subacute onset. Thunderclap headaches not typical of PACNS.

- **CNS complications** – Transient ischemic attacks, cerebral infarction, multifocal strokes, paraparesis, quadriparesis, hemiparesis, ataxia, seizures, aphasia, and visual field defects.

- **Cognitive function** – Decreased cognitive function or fluctuating levels of consciousness are not uncommon.

- **Differential diagnosis** – PACNS must be distinguished from the reversible cerebral vasoconstriction syndrome (RCVS). RCVS is not a true form of vasculitis but rather is induced by a variety of insults leading to vasospasm. Distinguishing these two conditions is critical because RCVS is much more common and has a dramatically different approach to therapy.

Cogan's Syndrome

- **Sensorineural hearing loss** – Bilateral. Often recurrent, progressive, and profound.

- **Ocular** – Non-syphilitic interstitial keratitis, scleritis, or uveitis are the most common eye manifestations.

- **Systemic** – Headache, fever, arthralgia, and vasculitis, with or without aortitis.

Erythema Elevatum Diutinum (EED)

- **Cutaneous lesions** – Purple, red, or brown plaques that occur over the extensor surfaces of joints and often have an annular or nodular appearance.

- **Comorbidity** – May occur in association with infectious diseases.

Diagnosis

PACNS

Early diagnosis is critical to prevent serious CNS morbidity.

- **Biopsy** – The most specific diagnostic procedure, but the sensitivity is only approximately 75%.

- **Cerebral angiogram** – Angiographic findings of vascular narrowing and dilatation are not specific for PACNS. RCVS can mimic PACNS perfectly on angiogram. Sensitivity of angiogram in PACNS is also low (~40–50%), because the size of blood vessels involved is often too small to be detected by angiogram.

- **Cerebral spinal fluid (CSF)** – Abnormal in 80–90% of cases of PACNS, but usually normal in RCVS. CSF findings in PACNS are characterized by a modest pleocytosis and elevated protein levels.

- **Magnetic resonance imaging** – Most common findings are multiple, bilateral, supratentorial infarctions distributed in the cortex, deep white matter and/or leptomeninges. Strokes, particularly multifocal ones, are uncommon in RCVS.

- **Exclude CNS infection** – CSF analysis should include appropriate stains, cultures, and serologic tests to exclude infections.

- **Progressive multifocal symptoms** – Occurrence of these symptoms over time in a younger patient should suggest the possibility of PACNS.

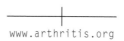

www.arthritis.org

Cogan's Syndrome

A multidisciplinary team (rheumatologist, otolaryngologist, and ophthalmologist) is required.

- **Onset** – Typically in third or fourth decade, with men and women affected equally.

- **Vestibular testing** – Shows bilateral cochlear dysfunction, helping to distinguish Cogan's from Ménière's syndrome.

EED

- **Exclude** – Neutrophilic dermatoses, primarily Sweet's syndrome.

Treatment

PACNS

- **Aggressive therapy** – High-dose glucocorticoids and a cytotoxic agent.

Cogan's Syndrome

- **Glucocorticoids** – Topically for anterior eye disease and systemically for audiovestibular manifestations, unremitting ocular disease, or when the disorder is complicated by vasculitis or significant systemic manifestations.

EED

Therapy of early lesions has a higher likelihood of success than treatment of long-established disease.

- **Comorbid conditions** – Treatment of any associated disorder may benefit EED.

- **Dapsone** – 100 mg/day may be successful.

Kawasaki's Disease

Kawasaki's disease (KD), once known as mucocutaneous lymph node syndrome, is a systemic inflammatory disorder of children (generally under the age of 6 years). KD is accompanied by vasculitis and a risk of coronary artery aneurysms.

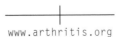

www.arthritis.org

Clinical Features

- **Principal criteria** – Fever lasting ≥4 days; bilateral non-purulent conjunctival injection; changes of the lips and oral cavity (including dry, fissured lips, strawberry tongue, diffuse reddening of the oropharyngeal mucosa); polymorphous rash primarily on the trunk; acute non-purulent swelling of a cervical lymph node to >1.5 cm; and changes of the peripheral extremities (including reddening of palms and soles, indurative edema of hands and feet, and membranous desquamation from the fingertips).

Diagnosis

- **American Heart Association (AHA) guidance** – To improve the treatment with intravenous immunoglobulin (IVIG), the AHA issued guidelines for the diagnosis of KD.

AHA Guidelines for Diagnosis of Kawasaki's Disease

Expanded epidemiologic case definition includes fever of ≥4 days and ≥4 principal criteria without other explanation OR fever and <4 principal criteria if coronary artery abnormalities are detected by echocardiogram or coronary angiography.

An echocardiogram should be performed in any patient ≤6 months of age if fever persists ≥7 days without other explanation and with laboratory measures of inflammation, even in the absence of any principal clinical criteria.

Laboratory parameters to help with diagnosis and determine disease severity: CRP ≥3.0 mg/dl, ESR ≥40 mm/h, albumin ≤3.0 g/dl, anemia for age, ↑ ALT, platelets after 7 days ≥450,000, WBC ≥15,000, urine microscopy ≥10 WBC/high-powered field.

ALT, alanine aminotransferase; CRP, C-reactive protein; ESR, erythrocyte sedimentation rate; WBC, white blood cell count.
Reproduced with permission from Pediatrics 2004; 114: 1708–1733. Copyright © 2004 by the AAP. And from Circulation 2004; 110: 2747–2771.

Treatment

- **Salicylates** – Potential for impedance of aspirin absorption caused by vasculitic involvement of the GI tract, therefore aspirin use must be monitored carefully.

- **IVIG** – In combination with aspirin. Early use of IVIG has been shown to prevent coronary artery aneurysms.

- **Glucocorticoids** – Role is controversial.

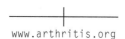

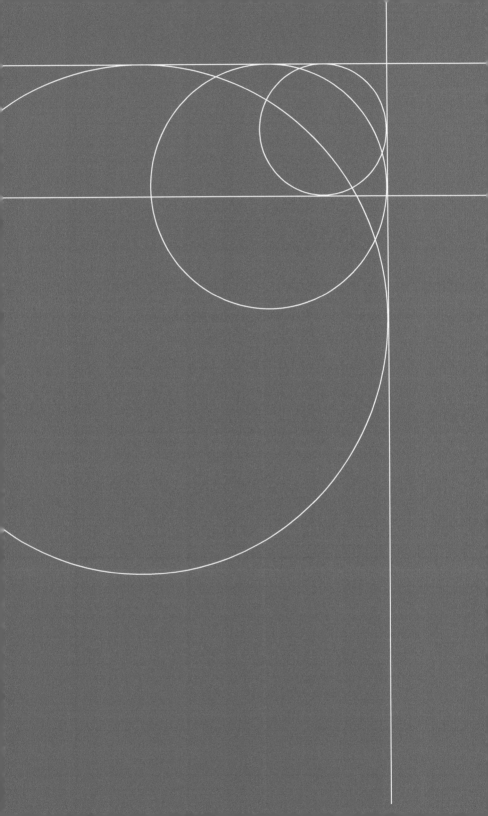

24 BEHÇET'S SYNDROME

Behçet's syndrome (BS) is a chronic inflammatory disorder of unknown cause.

Clinical Features

- **Onset** – Mean age 25–30 years.

- **Sex** – Equal distribution in Eastern Mediterranean countries, the Middle East, and East Asia. Females more commonly affected in Japan, Korea, and Western countries.

- **Ulcers** – Oral ulcers are the first and most prominent feature of BS. Genital and perianal ulcers also occur.

- **Pathergy** – Reflects neutrophil hyperreactivity and is highly specific for BS.

- **Skin lesions** – Erythema nodosum, pseudofolliculitis, papulopustular lesions, or acneform nodules can occur.

- **Ocular inflammation** – Typically anterior uveitis associated with a hypopyon, panuveitis with posterior chamber involvement and retinal vasculitis, and associated complications.

- **Cerebral venous thrombosis** – Patients usually present with symptoms of raised intracranial pressure: headache, visual obscurations, and papilledema.

- **Central nervous system (CNS) involvement** – Aseptic meningitis or parenchymal lesions can result in focal or diffuse brain dysfunction. Focal or multifocal nervous system involvement reflects the predilection of BS for diencephalon, midbrain, and brainstem. Closely mimics multiple sclerosis.

- **Deep venous thrombosis (DVT)** – The most common large vascular lesion.

- **Arterial complications** – Stenoses, occlusions, and aneurysms occur in the systemic circulation or the pulmonary arterial bed. The risk of aneurysm rupture is high.

- **Gastrointestinal (GI)** – Symptoms include melena and abdominal pain. GI tract inflammation can mimic inflammatory bowel disease (IBD).

- **Arthritis** – Intermittent, symmetric oligoarthritis of the knees, ankles, hands, or wrists; arthralgia is also common.

- **Epididymitis** – Occurs in 5% of patients with BS.

Laboratory Features

- **Acute-phase reactants** – May be normal or may be increased, particularly in patients with large-vessel vasculitis.

- **Human leukocyte antigen (HLA)-B51** – Associated with BS in areas of high prevalence and in patients with ocular disease.

Diagnosis

- **Pathergy** – The sensitivity of the test is lower in Western countries than in Silk Road countries, but a positive test adds great support for the diagnosis of BS.

- **Aphthosis** – Suggests BS when found in association with other disorders associated with large vessel disease or acute CNS infarction.

- **CNS symptoms** – The clinical combination of stroke, aseptic meningitis with cerebrospinal fluid pleocytosis, and mucocutaneous lesions is highly suggestive of BS.

- **Differential diagnosis** – The differential diagnosis of BS is shown in the table.

- **Exclude other systemic disorders** – IBD, sprue, cyclic neutropenia or other hematologic disorders, herpes simplex infection, and acquired immune deficiency syndrome may cause lesions similar to BS.

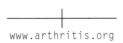

- **Exclude other disorders responsible for orogenital/ocular syndromes** – Including erythema multiforme, mucous membrane pemphigoid, and the vulvovaginal–gingival form of erosive lichen planus.

- **Exclude reactive arthritis** – The mucocutaneous lesions associated with reactive arthritis are painless and do not cause deep ulcerations, and the uveitis is usually limited to the anterior chamber, in contrast to the characteristic panuveitis of BS.

- **Exclude Crohn's disease** – Granuloma formation in intestinal lesions is not typical in BS. In Crohn's disease, the iritis is typically confined to the anterior chamber. Genital ulcerations and CNS disease are rare in Crohn's disease.

International Study Group Criteria for Behçet's syndrome

Recurrent oral ulceration	Minor aphthous, major aphthous, or herpetiform ulceration observed by physician or patient, which has recurred ≥3 times in one 12-month period[a]
Plus any two from:	
Recurrent genital ulceration	Aphthous ulceration or scarring, observed by physician or patient[a]
Eye lesions	Anterior uveitis, posterior uveitis, or cells in vitreous on slit lamp examination; or retinal vasculitis observed by ophthalmologist
Skin lesions	Erythema nodosum observed by physician or patient, pseudofolliculitis, or papulopustular lesions; or acneform nodules observed by physician in post-adolescent patients not receiving glucocorticoid treatment[a]
Positive pathergy test	Read by physician at 24–48 hours

[a] Findings only applicable in the absence of other clinical explanations.
Reprinted from the Lancet, Volume 335, by the International Study Group for Behçet's Disease. pp. 1078–1080. Copyright © 1990, with permission from Elsevier.

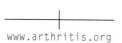

Treatment

- **Glucocorticoids** – Aphthous lesions are treated with topical or intralesional glucocorticoids. Glucocorticoids can be used to suppress acute episodes of inflammation. Short courses of prednisone are useful in the management of mucocutaneous disease in some patients.

- **Colchicine** – Frequently used but data surrounding efficacy unclear. GI intolerance can occur at higher doses.

- **Thalidomide** – Effective for mucocutaneous lesions, but toxicity is a major concern.

- **Glucocorticoid combination therapy** – With immunosuppressive agents for severe disease. Pulmonary arterial aneurysms may respond to the combination of prednisone and cyclophosphamide. Cerebral venous thrombosis is treated with anticoagulation and glucocorticoids. The treatment of Budd–Chiari syndrome includes anticoagulants and immunosuppressive medications.

- **Cyclosporine and azathioprine** – Monotherapy or in combination to treat uveitis. Azathioprine can have a beneficial effect on mucosal ulcers, arthritis, DVT, and long-term prognosis.

- **Tumor necrosis factor (TNF) inhibitors** – TNF inhibitors have largely supplanted alkylating agents such as cyclophosphamide and chlorambucil for the treatment of severe eye disease, particularly posterior uveitis. Can also be highly effective for CNS disease.

25 ADULT STILL'S DISEASE

Adult Still's disease is a systemic rheumatic disease characterized by high spiking fever, arthritis, and rash.

Clinical Features

- **High, spiking fever** – The initial symptom, usually in the evening.
- **Arthralgia, arthritis** – Joint complaints in virtually all patients.
- **Myalgia** – Common.
- **Still's rash** – Rash is salmon pink, macular or maculopapular, frequently evanescent, and often occurs with the evening fever spike.

Laboratory Features

- **Erythrocyte sedimentation rate** – Elevated.
- **Leukocytosis** – White blood cell count is 15,000/mm^3 or higher.
- **Liver function abnormalities** – May be elevated in up to three-quarters of patients.
- **Autoantibodies** – Rheumatoid factor and antinuclear antibody negative.
- **Serum ferritin level** – Extreme elevations are not unusual.

Radiographic Features

- **Radiographic findings** – Nonspecific at presentation. With time, cartilage narrowing or erosion develops in most patients.

Diagnosis

- **Criteria** – The criteria of Cush et al. are a practical guide (see Table).
- **Note** – Most patients do not present with the full-blown syndrome. Fever is the most common initial manifestation, and other features develop over a period of weeks or, occasionally, months.

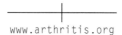

Criteria for the Diagnosis of Adult Still's Disease

A diagnosis of adult Still's disease requires the presence of all the following:
Fever ≥39°C (102.2°F)
Arthralgia or arthritis
Rheumatoid factor <1:80
Antinuclear antibody <1:100
In addition, any two of the following are required:
White blood cell count ≥15,000 cells/mm^3
Still's rash
Pleuritis or pericarditis
Hepatomegaly or splenomegaly or generalized lymphadenopathy

Reprinted from Cush JJ, Medsger TA, Jr, Christy WC, Herbert DC, Cooperstein LA. Adult-onset Still's disease. Clinical course and outcome. Arthritis Rheum 1987; 30: 186–194. Copyright © 1987 American College of Rheumatology. Reproduced with permission of John Wiley & Sons, Inc.

- **Exclude** – The differential diagnosis list is large.

Treatment

Acute Disease

- **NSAIDs** – NSAIDs are the first line of therapy, and response may be slow.

- **Liver function** – Monitoring is mandatory for patients receiving NSAIDs, even after hospital discharge.

- **Glucocorticoids** – Used for patients whose disease fails to respond to NSAIDs, and those with severe disease. Severe disease includes pericardial tamponade, myocarditis, severe pneumonitis, intravascular coagulopathy, and rising values on liver function tests during NSAID treatment.

Differential Diagnosis of Adult Still's Disease

Granulomatous disorders
Sarcoidosis Idiopathic granulomatosis hepatitis Crohn's disease
Vasculitis
Serum sickness Polyarteritis nodosa Wegener's granulomatosis Thrombotic thrombocytopenia purpura Takayasu's arteritis
Infection
Viral infection (e.g. hepatitis B, rubella, parvovirus, Coxsackie virus, Epstein-Barr, cytomegalovirus, HIV) Subacute bacterial endocarditis Chronic meningococcemia Gonococcemia Tuberculosis Rheumatic fever
Malignancy
Leukemia Lymphoma Angioblastic lymphadenopathy
Connective-tissue disease
Systemic lupus erythematosus Mixed connective-tissue disease

Chronic Disease

- **Arthritis control** – Weekly methotrexate has been used to control both chronic arthritis and chronic systemic disease. Anakinra, an antagonist of the interleukin-1 receptor, is employed in cases refractory to glucocorticoids and methotrexate.

- **Adjunct therapy** – Physical therapists, occupational therapists, psychologists, and arthritis support groups may be needed to care for individual patients.

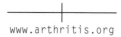

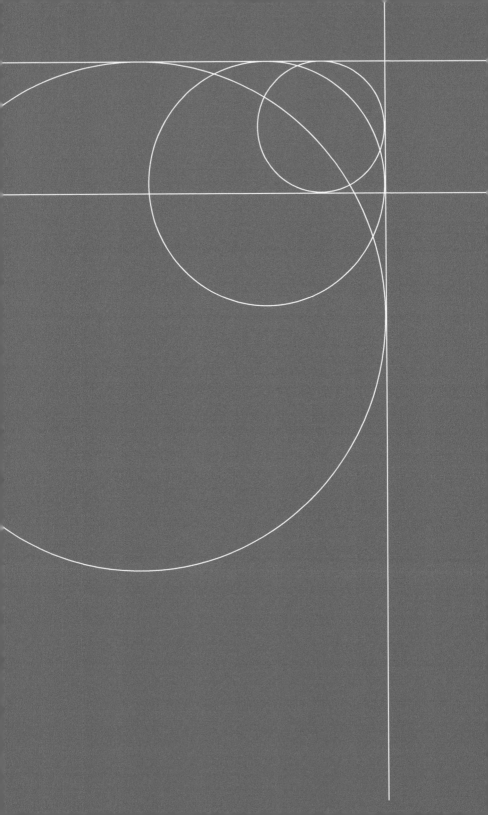

26 AUTOINFLAMMATORY DISORDERS/PERIODIC SYNDROMES

A group of diseases characterized by episodes of fever with serosal, synovial, and/or cutaneous inflammation. Most of these syndromes are hereditary, but some are idiopathic.

Clinical Features and Treatment

- **Hereditary periodic syndromes** – Systemic. See table for key clinical features of each type of syndrome. Hereditary periodic fever syndromes are now often termed "autoinflammatory syndromes." These disorders are generally caused by single gene mutations.

- **Idiopathic periodic syndromes** – Primarily affect joints and adjacent structures. Tend to affect both genders evenly. See table for key clinical features of each type of syndrome.

Hereditary Periodic Fever (Autoinflammatory) Syndromes

Feature	FMF	HIDS	TRAPS
Mode of inheritance	Autosomal recessive	Autosomal recessive	Autosomal dominant
Underlying gene	*MEFV*, encoding pyrin (marenostrin)	*MVK*, encoding mevalonate kinase	*TNFRS1A*, encoding p55 TNF receptor
Usual ethnicity	Turkish, Armenian, Arab, Jewish, Italian	Dutch, other North European	Any ethnicity
Duration of attacks	12–72 hours	3–7 days	Days to weeks
Abdominal pain	Sterile peritonitis, constipation	Severe pain, vomiting, diarrhea, rarely peritonitis	Peritonitis, diarrhea, or constipation
Pleural involvement	Common	Rare	Common
Arthropathy	Monarthritis; rarely protracted arthritis in knee or hip	Arthralgia, symmetric polyarthritis	Arthritis in large joints, arthralgia
Cutaneous involvement	Erysipeloid erythema on lower leg, ankle, foot	Diffuse maculopapular rash, urticaria	Migratory rash with underlying myalgia
Ocular involvement	Rare	Uncommon	Periorbital edema conjunctivitis
Neurologic involvement	Rarely aseptic meningitis	Headache	Controversial
Lymphatic involvement	Splenomegaly, occasional lymphadenopathy	Painful cervical lymphadenopathy in children	Splenomegaly, occasional lymphadenopathy
Vasculitis	HSP, polyarteritis nodosa	Cutaneous vasculitis common, rarely HSP	HSP, lymphocytic vasculitis
Systemic amyloidosis	Depends on *MEFV* and *SAA* genotypes; more common in Middle East	Rare	Occurs in 15%; risk increased with cysteine mutations
Treatment	Daily colchicine prophylaxis	Anti-TNF, statins investigational	Glucocorticoids, etanercept

FCAS, familial cold autoinflammatory syndrome; FMF, familial Mediterranean fever; HIDS, hyperimmunoglobulinemia D with periodic fever syndrome; HSP, Henoch–Schönlein purpura; MWS, Muckle–Wells syndrome.

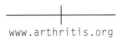

FCAS	MWS	NOMID (CINCA)
Autosomal dominant	Autosomal dominant	Autosomal dominant
CIAS1, encoding cryopyrin (NALP3)	*CIAS1*, encoding cryopyrin	*CIAS1*, encoding cryopyrin (NALP3)
Mostly European	Mostly European	Any ethnicity
12–24 hours	2–3 days	Continuous, with flares
Nausea	Abdominal pain, vomiting, diarrhea	Can occur
Not seen	Rare	Rare
Polyarthralgia	Polyarthralgia, oligoarthritis, clubbing	Epiphyseal overgrowth, contractures, intermittent or chronic arthritis, clubbing
Cold-induced urticarial rash	Urticaria-like rash	Urticaria-like rash
Conjunctivitis	Conjunctivitis, episcleritis	Progressive visual loss, uveitis, conjunctivitis
Headache	Sensorineural deafness	Headache, sensorineural deafness, chronic aseptic meningitis, mental retardation
Not seen	Rare	Hepatosplenomegaly, lymphadenopathy
Not seen	Not seen	Occasional
Rare	Occurs in ~25% patients	May develop in some, usually in adulthood
Anakinra	Anakinra	Anakinra

NOMID (CINCA), neonatal-onset multisystem inflammatory disease (chronic infantile neurologic cutaneous and articular syndrome); TNF, tumor necrosis factor; TRAPS, tumor necrosis periodic factor receptor-associated syndrome.

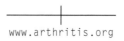

Idiopathic Periodic Syndromes

Feature	Palindromic rheumatism	Intermittent hydrarthrosis	Eosinophilic synovitis
Onset	Mean age of 45 years	20–50 years of age	20–50 years of age
Attacks	Last ~2 days; monarticular arthritis or periarticular soft-tissue inflammation	Last 3–5 days; monarticular arthritis, large effusions	Last 1–2 weeks; monoarthritis triggered by trauma
Joints involved	MCPs, PIPs, wrists, shoulders, MTPs, ankles	Knee to hip, ankle, elbow	Knee, MTP
Associated conditions	Familial aggregation with RA	Episodes may coincide with menses; heterozygous MEFV mutations?	Personal or family history of atopy, dermatographism
Prognosis	~50% persistent palindromic rheumatism, ~33% develop RA	Attacks often occur at predictable intervals; sometimes spontaneous remissions	Self-limited episodes; benign prognosis
Treatment	Injectable gold, antimalarials, sulfasalazine, glucocorticoids, synovectomy	NSAIDs, colchicine, intra-articular glucocorticoids, synovectomy	Symptomatic

MCP, metacarpophalangeal joint; MTP, metatarsophalangeal joint; NSAID, nonsteriodal anti-inflammatory drug; PIP, proximal interphalangeal joint; RA, rheumatoid arthritis.

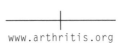

27 LESS COMMON ARTHROPATHIES

Hematologic and Malignant Disorders

Hemophilia and Musculoskeletal Symptoms

- **Recurrent hemarthrosis** – Primary clinical manifestation.

- **Causes** – Repeated intra-articular bleeding and excessive iron deposition within joints.

- **Radiographs** – Often show increased periarticular soft-tissue swelling in the synovium. Widening or premature fusion of the epiphyses, enlargement of the femoral and humeral intercondylar notches, "squaring" of the inferior patella, expansion of the radial head at the elbow, and secondary osteoarthritis may occur in later stages.

- **Treatment of acute hemarthrosis** – Ice packs and prompt administration of factor VIII, joint aspiration, and short-term use of glucocorticoids.

- **Treatment of chronic hemarthrosis** – Nonsteroidal anti-inflammatory drugs (NSAIDs; not aspirin), physical therapy, surgical or arthroscopic synovectomy.

Sickle Cell Disease and Musculoskeletal Symptoms

- **Sickle cell arthropathy** – Caused by microvascular ischemia and synovial infarctions.

- **Recurrent painful crises** – Mainly affect the juxta-articular areas of long bones, joints, spine, and ribs.

- **Osteonecrosis** – Mostly affects the femoral or humeral heads, but may affect multiple joints. Total replacement arthroplasty is recommended for those with advanced secondary osteoarthritis.

- **Dactylitis** – Acute, painful, non-pitting swelling of hands and feet.

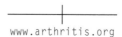

www.arthritis.org

- **Osteomyelitis** – Caused by ischemic bone infarction and impaired immunity. Salmonella organisms are often the etiologic agents.

- **Painful crisis prevention** – Avoidance of stress, alcohol, overexertion, swimming, and high altitudes.

- **Painful crisis treatment** – Acetaminophen, NSAIDs, codeine, oxycodone, or morphine, depending on severity.

Thalassemia and Musculoskeletal Symptoms

- **Musculoskeletal manifestations** – Only associated with beta-thalassemia major and include osteoporosis with wide medullary spaces, coarse trabeculae, pathologic fractures, epiphyseal deformities, and leg shortening.

Malignant Disease and Musculoskeletal Symptoms

- **Mechanisms** – Direct tumor invasion of bones and joints (skeletal metastases, metastatic carcinomatous arthritis, leukemic synovitis, and lymphomatous arthritis); hemorrhage into the joint (leukemia); secondary gout (leukemia, polycythemia, lymphoma, myeloma, carcinoma); and through remote, non-metastatic effects of the tumor (paraneoplastic syndromes), such as hypertrophic osteoarthropathy.

Rheumatic Disease and Endocrinopathies

- **Glucocorticoid excess** – Cushing's syndrome or exogenous administration can cause musculoskeletal complications such as osteoporosis.

- **Glucocorticoid deficiency** – Addison's disease can cause myalgias, arthralgias, and flexion contractures.

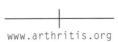

Rheumatologic Manifestations of Endocrinopathies

Endocrine disorder	Rheumatologic manifestations
Diabetes mellitus	Syndromes of limited joint mobility: diabetic hand syndrome (diabetic cheiroarthropathy); adhesive capsulitis (frozen shoulder, periarthritis); trigger finger (flexor tenosynovitis); Dupuytren's contractures Osteoporosis Diffuse idiopathic skeletal hyperostosis Neuropathies: neuropathic arthritis (Charcot joints, diabetic osteoarthropathy); carpal tunnel syndrome; diabetic amyotrophy; reflex sympathetic dystrophy (multiple synonyms) Various other neuropathies Diabetic muscle infarction
Hyperthyroidism	Osteoporosis Myopathy Periarthritis Acropachy
Hypothyroidism	Arthralgias Symmetrical polyarthritis Joint laxity Carpal tunnel syndrome Chondrocalcinosis and pseudogout Hyperuricemia and gout Myopathy
Hyperparathyroidism	Osteoporosis Osteitis fibrosa cystica Erosive arthritis Joint laxity Chondrocalcinosis and pseudogout Hyperuricemia and gout Myopathy
Hypoparathyroidism	Ectopic calcification Myopathy
Acromegaly	Articular: arthralgias; bursal enlargement; osteoarthritis; joint laxity; cartilage hypertrophy and degeneration; pseudogout (possibly); tendinous and capsular calcification Bone: back pain; osteoporosis; bone hypertrophy and resorption Neuromuscular: myopathy and muscle hypertrophy; compression neuropathy, particularly carpal tunnel syndrome; ischemic neuropathy Miscellaneous: Raynaud's phenomenon

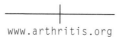

www.arthritis.org

Hyperlipidemia and Musculoskeletal Clinical Features

Phenotype	Lipoprotein abnormality	Lipid abnormality
I	Chylomicrons increased	Markedly increased triglycerides
IIa	LDL increased	Increased cholesterol
IIb	LDL and VLDL increased	Increased cholesterol and triglycerides
III	Chylomicrons and VLDL remnants increased	Increased cholesterol; increased to markedly increased triglycerides
IV	VLDL increased	Increased triglycerides
V	Chylomicrons and VLDL increased	Increased cholesterol, markedly increased triglycerides

LDL, low-density lipoprotein, VLDL, very low-density lipoprotein.
Modified from Fredrickson DS, Levy RI, Lees RS. N Engl J Med 1967; 276: 34–42.

Hypolipoproteinemia and Arthritis

- **Radiographs** – Can include calcifications within the xanthomas, or even periarticular cortical erosions. Osseous xanthomas have the appearance of well-defined, round or oval lucencies.

- **Tendinous xanthomas** – Pathological examination reveals infiltrates of foam cells that seem to be macrophages congested with remnants of ingested circulating lipoproteins.

- **Articular disease** – Controversial. An episodic, acute, migratory inflammatory arthritis occurs in up to 50% of homozygotes with type II hyperlipoproteinemia, which primarily affects large peripheral joints, such as knees and ankles. Acute mono- or oligoarthritis can be seen in familial hypercholesterolemia.

- **Cholesterol crystals** – Result in gout and can be associated with hypertriglyceridemia in types I, IV, and V hyperlipoproteinemia.

- **Treatment** – NSAIDs can be helpful; treatment of underlying dyslipidemia and surgical excision (especially of Achilles tendon) can be beneficial.

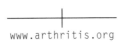

Musculoskeletal manifestation
Eruptive xanthomas
Tendinous, tuberous xanthomas; migratory, episodic polyarthritis; Achilles tendinitis
Tendinous, tuberous xanthomas; migratory, episodic polyarthritis; Achilles tendinitis
Tendinous, tuberous and plane xanthomas
Eruptive tendinous and tuberous xanthomas; arthralgias
Eruptive xanthomas

Neuropathic Arthropathy

- **Monarthritis** – Neuropathic arthropathy typically presents as an acute or subacute monarthritis with swelling, erythema, and variable amounts of pain in the affected joint.

- **Prominent clinical features** – The two most consistent features are the presence of a significant sensory deficit and pain that is less than expected for the amount of joint destruction.

- **Diabetic foot** – Midfoot involvement is particularly common.

- **Differential diagnosis** – Includes osteomyelitis and other deep tissue infections, fracture, gout, calcium pyrophosphate dihydrate deposition (CPPD) disease, Milwaukee shoulder/knee syndrome, osteonecrosis, and osteoarthritis. A combined approach using multiple imaging techniques with or without bone cultures is often necessary to differentiate infection from neuropathic arthropathy.

- **Plain radiographs** – Extremely helpful in making the diagnosis.

- **Early features** – Demineralization, joint space narrowing, and osteophyte formation.

www.arthritis.org

- **Established disease** – Bone fragmentation, periarticular debris formation, and joint subluxation.

- **Treatment goals** – Improve pain, joint stability, and alignment, and prevent or treat overlying skin ulceration. Prevention is probably the best therapy – control blood sugar levels and treat any minor trauma to foot or ankle to prevent development of neuropathic arthropathy.

- **Joint immobilization** – Effective therapy usually achieved by casts, braces, orthotics, and restricted weight-bearing.

- **Prevention** – Good control of diabetes, and prompt attention to diabetic foot or ankle trauma.

Dermatologic Disorders

Many rheumatologic diseases have prominent cutaneous findings.

Neutrophilic Dermatoses

- **Sweet's syndrome** – Often associated with malignancy, inflammatory disease, infection, and drugs, and characterized by painful erythematous plaques which can be treated with glucocorticoids or immunosuppressive agents.

- **Pyroderma gangrenosum** – Diagnosed by exclusion, this ulcerative skin disease has four clinical variants: classical, atypical, peristomal and mucosal. Prednisone, dapsone, cyclosporine, and tumor necrosis factor inhibitors can be effective.

- **Other dermatoses** – Neutrophilic dermatosis of the dorsal hands; rheumatoid neutrophilic dermatosis which is an unusual complication of rheumatoid arthritis; and bowel-associated dermatosis–arthritis syndrome which is now very rare.

Panniculitides

- **Erythema nodosum** – Commonly triggered by upper respiratory tract or lung infection, it is characterized by red, tender, subcutaneous nodules often on the anterior leg, and can occur with joint inflammation. Support, elevation, and NSAIDs appear effective.

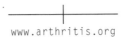

- **Weber–Christian disease** – Characterized by recurrent, often multiple, tender subcutaneous nodules with accompanying fever, but controversy exists as to whether it is a primary disorder or a complication of an underlying illness.

- **Lupus panniculitis** – A rare manifestation of systemic lupus erythematosus.

- **Lipodermatosclerosis** – Characterized by tender, subcutaneous nodules most often over the medial malleolus, accompanied by hyperpigmentation, telangiectases, tortuous veins, edema, and a woody induration. Support stockings are an effective therapy.

- **Calcifying panniculitis** – Most often occurs in people with renal failure.

- **Cytophagic histiocytic panniculitis** – Associated with an underlying lymphoma, manifests as tender subcutaneous nodules, fever, hepatosplenomegaly, pancytopenia, and serositis.

Sclerosing/Fibrosing Diseases

- **Localized scleroderma** – Differentiated from systemic sclerosis by the lack of Raynaud's phenomenon, sclerodactyly, and the absence of internal organ involvement.

- **Lichen sclerosus** – Linked to circulating antibodies directed against extracellular matrix protein 1, manifests by induration and superficial, atrophic, hypopigmented patches or plaques that resemble cigarette paper. Treated with potent glucocorticoids.

- **Scleromyxedema** – Characterized by a generalized papular and sclerodermatous eruption (often described as "waxy papules") of the head, neck, arms, and upper trunk.

- **Nephrogenic systemic fibrosis** – Characterized by a rapid onset of skin thickening and accompanied by a limited range of motion in patients with renal disease. A history of gadolinium administration for the performance of a magnetic resonance imaging study is the sine qua non of this condition.

Pustular Conditions

- **Generalized pustular psoriasis** – Localized to the palms and soles.

- **SAPHO syndrome** – Rare, and characterized by synovitis, acne, pustulosis of the palms and soles, hyperostosis of one of the bones of the chest wall, and sterile osteitis.

- **PAPA syndrome** – Characterized by sterile pyogenic arthritis, pyoderma gangrenosum, and acne. See chapter 26, Periodic (Auto-inflammatory) Syndromes.

- **Hidradenitis suppurativa** – A disorder of apocrine glands, which manifests by pustules and draining sinus tracts in the axilla, under the breasts, within inguinal folds, and on the buttocks. May be associated with Crohn's disease.

- **Acne fulminans** – A severe form of acne.

Other Dermatoses

- **Conditions with possible rheumatic consequences** – Scurvy, livedoid vasculopathy, granuloma annulare, cutaneous extravascular necrotizing granulomas, and lichen planus.

Hypertrophic Osteoarthropathy

Hypertrophic osteoarthropathy (HOA) is a syndrome characterized by excessive proliferation of skin and bone at the distal parts of the extremities.

Clinical Features

- **Clubbing** – Most conspicuous feature of HOA is a unique bulbous deformity of the tips of the digits. Develops as a result of edema and excessive collagen deposition.

- **Periostosis** – Evolves in an orderly manner, with symmetrical bone changes.

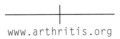

- **Bone pain** – Particularly affects those with pulmonary malignancies. Characteristically, this pain is incapacitating, deep-seated, and often more prominent in the legs.

- **Pachyderma** – Affects some people with primary HOA.

Diagnosis

- **Clubbing** – Most prominent feature.

- **Adjacent bone pain** – Pain not only in the joint, but also the adjacent bones, distinguishes HOA from inflammatory types of arthritis.

Radiographs

- **Mild periostosis** – Affects the distal parts of the lower extremities and then progresses in a centripetal fashion. Involves only few selected bones (usually the tibia and fibula) and is limited to the diaphysis, with a monolayer configuration.

- **Severe periostosis** – Affects all tubular bones, spreads to the metaphyses and epiphyses and generates irregular configurations.

- **Joint space** – Typically preserved, with no erosions or periarticular osteopenia.

- **Radionuclide bone scanning** – Sensitive method for demonstrating periosteal involvement.

Treatment

- **Analgesics or NSAIDs** – Effective at reducing painful manifestations.

- **Bisphosphonates** – Potent inhibitors of vascular endothelial growth factor (VEGF) – a protein believed to play an important role in HOA. Anecdotal evidence supports the use of bisphosphonates in this condition.

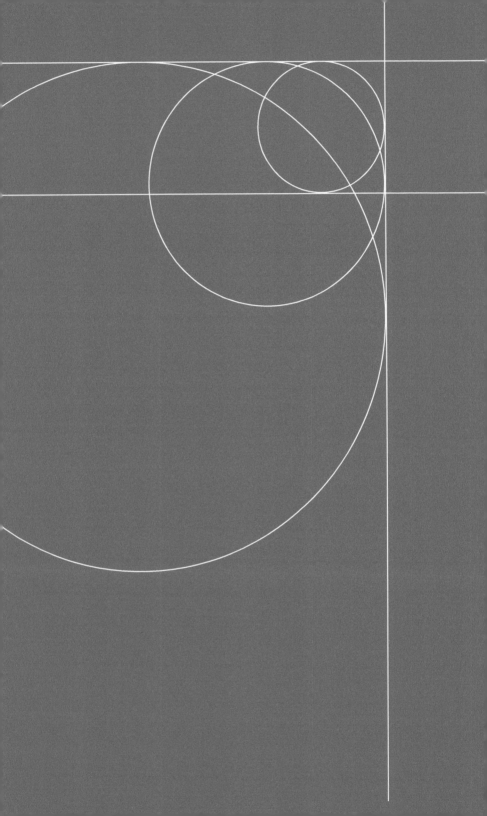

28 COMPLEX REGIONAL PAIN SYNDROME

Complex regional pain syndrome (CRPS) is a disorder of the musculoskeletal system that primarily relates to abnormal functioning of the sensory, sympathetic, and motor nerves.

Clinical Features

- **Onset** – May occur at any age, but most commonly between 40 and 60 years.

- **Trauma** – Precedes CRPS in approximately 50% of cases.

- **Other causes** – Medical disorders are the cause in about 25% of cases. These include diseases of the central nervous system or disorders of the peripheral nerves. Barbiturates and isoniazid, as well as pregnancy, metastatic tumors, and prolonged immobilization of a limb, are also associated with CRPS. About 25% of CRPS cases are idiopathic.

- **Distal involvement** – Patella, digit, hand, or foot are typically affected. The key symptom is pain that is out of proportion to any local tissue damage.

- **Pain** – The majority have persistent, spontaneous pain that is often described as having a tearing or burning quality. Lancinating pain occurs in one-third of cases, and activity-induced pain is present in all. Most severe discomfort and allodynia is present distally, but the majority of patients have abnormal tenderness of the entire quadrant of the involved limb. In about 25% of cases, the opposite limb also develops similar but less marked clinical features.

- **Abnormal cutaneous sensitivity** – Allodynia (whereby otherwise innocuous stimuli induce pain) and hyperalgesia (whereby pain perception is increased in response to a given painful stimulus).

- **Swelling** – Common, but usually diffuse and often associated with reticular or livedoid appearance over the skin of the involved area.

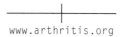

- **Muscle dysfunction** – Many develop peripheral weakness, proximal co-contraction and tightness, dystonia, spasm, tremor, or myoclonus. Tendon reflexes are usually normal or brisk.

- **Variable clinical pattern** – Changes in skin color (cyanotic, pale, or red), temperature, and sweating may occur.

Diagnosis

- **Early diagnosis** – There are no specific abnormal results to laboratory or imaging studies. Clinical features remain the most important contributors to diagnosis. Key clinical predictors for the problem are regional pain occurring in an emotional context, particularly after injury. Pain that seems out of proportion to the original injury, particularly when it becomes more diffuse and persistent, coupled with swelling and vasomotor changes, are the common early features.

Treatment

- **Early intervention** – Response to treatment in CRPS is unpredictable. Generally, earlier diagnosis and intervention result in better outcomes.

- **Multidisciplinary team** – Relevant family members and health professionals, which could include an occupational therapist, physiotherapist, psychologist, and physician.

- **Preventive strategies** – Identification of clinical situations common to CRPS:

  - **Early mobilization** – After myocardial infarction, cerebrovascular accident, hand surgery, or mild peripheral injury.

  - **Physical therapy** – Essential.

  - **Reassurance** – In the post-traumatic setting as part of routine treatment.

  - **Education** – Addressing anxiety and sleep disturbance with explanation. Patient education about the nature of the problem and the expected good prognosis are essential.

- **Exercise** – Programs that include hydrotherapy can be very helpful in mild CRPS. To achieve good exercise, adequate analgesia may be required.

- **Low-dose tricyclic medications** – Amitriptyline 25–50 mg.

- **Glucocorticoids** – Prednisone 25–50 mg per day over a few weeks with subsequent tapering of dose may be effective in early CRPS.

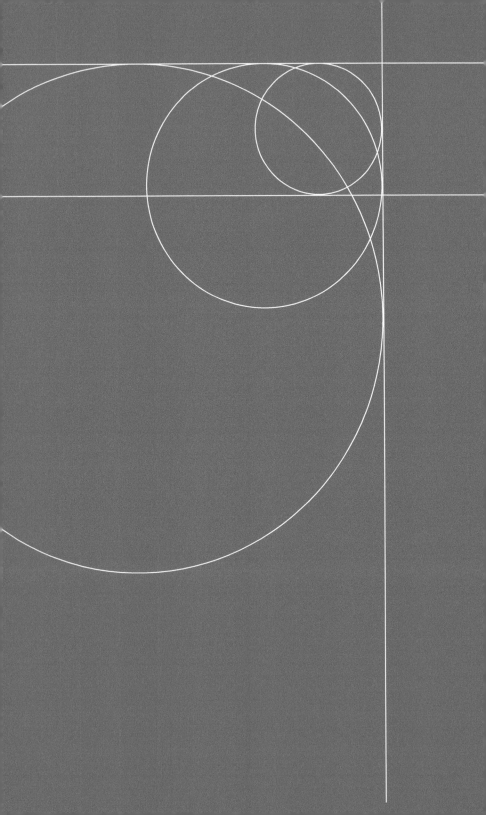

29 OSTEONECROSIS

Osteonecrosis (avascular necrosis) refers to a form of arthritis produced by death of a segment of bone adjacent to joints.

Clinical Features

- **Joints affected** – Can develop in any joint, but most commonly occurs in hips, knees, ankles, and shoulders.

- **Pain** – First clinical manifestation. Onset can be abrupt or insidious. Initially, pain is present only with movement, but later escalates to pain at rest.

- **Range of motion** – Progressive loss of joint motion as disease progresses.

- **Function** – Significant loss of function can occur as a result of pain and loss of range of movement.

Radiographic Features

- **Stages of disease** – Stages of disease progression are determined through radiographs and magnetic resonance imaging (MRI).

Diagnosis

- **Imaging** – Plain radiographs identify advanced disease but do not detect early stages. MRI is the diagnostic tool of choice for identifying early disease.

- **Glucocorticoids** – The higher the dose, the greater the likelihood of osteonecrosis.

- **Associated illnesses** – Other conditions associated with osteonecrosis are shown in the accompanying table.

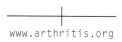

Staging in Osteonecrosis

Stage 0	Clinical manifestations absent; normal radiographs[a]
Stage I	Clinical manifestations present; normal radiographs[a]
Stage II	Areas of osteopenia and osteosclerosis in radiographs
Stage III	Early bone collapse manifested as the "crescent sign" (translucent subcortical bone delineates the area of dead bone)
Stage IV	Late bone collapse manifested as flattening of the femoral head, with or without joint incongruity

[a] Diagnosis made by magnetic resonance imaging.

Treatment

- **Conservative treatment** – Judicious use of analgesics, physical therapy to maintain muscle strength and prevent contractures, and assistive devices to facilitate ambulation.

- **Core decompression** – Important to consider in people with stage I or II osteonecrosis. The rationale is to reduce intraosseous pressure, reestablish blood supply, and allow living bone adjacent to dead bone to contribute to the reparative process.

- **Arthroplasty** – Patients with persistent, intractable pain and progressive functional loss should be considered for arthroplasty.

Diseases or Conditions Associated with Osteonecrosis

Trauma
- Hip dislocation
- Hip fracture
- Postarthroscopy

Connective-tissue disorders (CTDs)[a]
- Systemic lupus erythematosus
- Rheumatoid arthritis
- Systemic vasculitis
- Antiphospholipid antibody syndrome
- Other CTDs

Hematologic disorders
- Sickle cell disease
- Sickle cell-C disease
- Thalassemia minor
- Clotting disorders[b]

Infiltrative disorders
- Gaucher's disease
- Solid tumors

Metabolic disorders
- Gout

Disorders associated with fat necrosis
- Pancreatitis
- Pancreatic carcinoma

Embolism
- Decompression sickness

Glucocorticoids (exogenous and endogenous)
- Asthma
- Aplastic anemia
- Leukemias and lymphomas
- Celiac disease
- Inflammatory bowel disease
- Cushing's syndrome
- Organ transplantation
- Intra-articular, pulse intravenous, and enteral administration

Gastrointestinal disorders
- Inflammatory bowel disease[a]

Cytotoxic agents
- Vinblastine
- Vincristine
- Cisplatin (intra-arterial)
- Cyclophosphamide
- Methotrexate
- Bleomycin
- 5-Fluorouracil

Alcohol

Radiation

Pregnancy

Idiopathic[c]

[a] May occur independent of glucocorticoid use.
[b] Intravascular coagulation associated with infections included.
[c] No associated disorders or precipitating factors recognized.

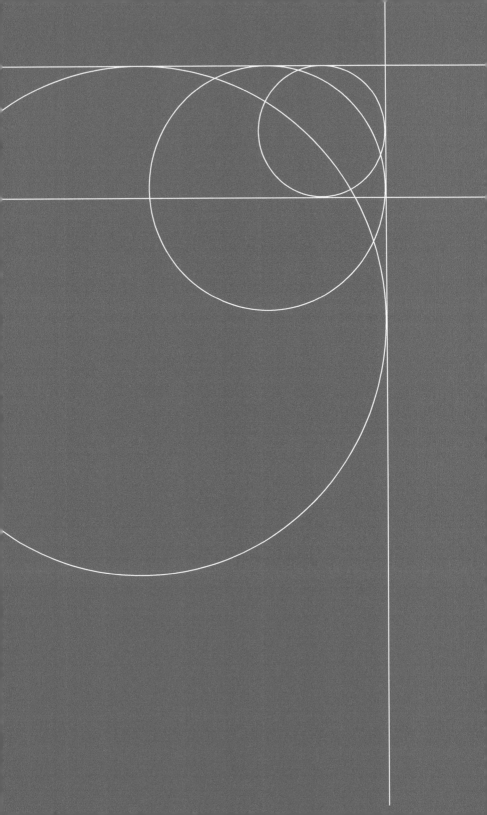

30 PAGET'S DISEASE

Paget's disease is a localized disorder of bone remodeling, in which the production of bone is disorganized, leading to thickened, weak, and often hypervascular bone. The cellular dysfunction in Paget's disease is centered on the osteoclast.

Clinical Features

- **Sites affected** – Pelvis, spine, and femur most commonly. Involvement of the skull and tibia also is common.

- **Asymptomatic** – Paget's disease frequently is asymptomatic, and the diagnosis often is made as an incidental finding on X-rays.

- **Presenting features** – Pain, bony deformity, or neurologic manifestations.

- **Joint pain** – Although Paget's disease classically spares joints, periarticular disease may result in significant pain in the hips, knees, or spine.

- **Bony deformities** – Uncommon, but highly specific for Paget's disease.

- **Skull abnormalities** – Narrowing of neural foramina may produce neurologic sequelae, the most common being hearing loss.

- **Complications** – Risk for excessive bleeding after a fracture and the development of bony malignancy.

Laboratory Features

- **Bone alkaline phosphatase** – The most effective method for monitoring disease activity and assessing the effectiveness of therapy.

- **Urinary hydroxyproline** – Measure of bone resorption, typically elevated.

- **Collagen cross-links** – Measure of bone resorption, typically elevated.

Radiographic Features

- **Bony lysis** – Classic radiographic finding, reflecting increased osteoclast activity.

- **Sclerosis** – Classic radiographic finding, reflecting increased osteoblast activity.

- **Bone thickening** – Highly characteristic of Paget's disease.

- **Flame-shaped lytic lesion** – Seen in long bones, highly characteristic.

- **Bone scans** – Can help determine the extent of bony involvement, but should not be used to make the diagnosis.

Diagnosis

- **Diagnosis** – Made by radiographs, routine laboratory testing, or both.

Treatment

- **Bisphosphonates** – Current first-line of therapy. Short, two to three month course is highly effective and well tolerated.

- **Treatment criteria** – Patients who are symptomatic, at risk for complications, and with markedly elevated levels of alkaline phosphatase.

- **Monitor** – Alkaline phosphatase levels should be monitored during bisphosphonate therapy, and subsequently, at three to six month intervals. If alkaline phosphate levels rise, an additional course of bisphosphonates often is effective in controlling disease activity.

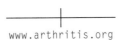

www.arthritis.org

31 OSTEOPOROSIS

Osteoporosis is a disease characterized by low bone mass and an increased risk of fractures.

Clinical Features

- **Sites affected** – Spine, hip, and wrists are most commonly affected.

- **Acute symptoms** – An osteoporotic fracture is typically associated with intense, localized pain, periarticular muscle spasm, and reduced joint motion.

- **Vertebral fractures** – May be completely asymptomatic and associated only with a loss of height, and progressive kyphosis (dowager's hump). Vertebral fractures in the lumbar spine result in progressive flattening of the lordotic curve, and scoliosis may develop.

Laboratory Features

- **Low bone mass** – The strongest predictor of future fracture is bone mass.

- **Fracture risk** – Risk increases with decreasing bone mineral density (BMD) levels.

- **Bone densitometry** – Densitometry required to measure BMD, and to identify and follow individuals at risk for fracture. Bone densitometry is recommended in: a) all postmenopausal women who present with a fracture; b) in postmenopausal women under the age of 65 who have one or more risk factors for osteoporosis; and c) all women over 65 years of age regardless of risk factors.

- **Measurement devices** – Devices are categorized by whether they measure the central skeleton (spine and hip) or the peripheral skeleton (finger, heel, tibia, and wrist/forearm).

- **DEXA** – Central device most commonly used. Central DEXA scans have software to measure total body bone mass, body composition, and vertebral morphometry.

Diagnosis

- **WHO criteria** – In 1994, the World Health Organization provided criteria for the diagnosis of normal bone mass, low bone mass or osteopenia, and osteoporosis. The WHO criteria for the spine, hip, and wrist apply only to White postmenopausal women.

World Health Organization Criteria for the Diagnosis of Osteoporosis

Normal:	BMC or BMD not more than 1 standard deviation below peak adult bone mass T-score > –1
Osteopenia:	BMC or BMD that lies between 1 and 2.5 standard deviations below peak adult bone mass T-score between –1 and –2.5
Osteoporosis:	BMC or BMD value more than 2.5 standard deviations below peak adult bone mass T-score ≤ –2.5
Severe osteoporosis:	BMC or BMD value more than 2.5 standard deviations below peak adult bone mass and the presence of one or more fragility fractures T-score ≤ –2.5 plus fragility fracture

World Health Organization criteria for the diagnosis of osteoporosis based on bone mineral content (BMC) or bone mineral density (BMD) measurements. These criteria can be applied to either the central or peripheral skeletal measurement sites.

Treatment

- **Goals** – The main goal of osteoporosis management is the prevention of fractures.

- **Guidelines** – National Osteoporosis Foundation guidelines for diagnosis and treatment of osteoporosis are shown.

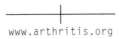

Recommendations for Diagnosis and Treatment of Osteoporosis

1. Urge postmenopausal women to consider their risk of osteoporosis. Osteoporosis is a "silent" risk factor for fracture, just as hypertension is for stroke.

2. Implement a system in your office whereby at-risk women have their skeletal health addressed and recorded at every visit.

3. Evaluate for osteoporosis all postmenopausal women who present with fractures. Use bone mineral density (BMD) testing to confirm the diagnosis and determine disease severity.

4. Recommend BMD testing to postmenopausal women under age 65 who have one or more risk factors, other than menopause, for osteoporotic fractures.

5. Recommend BMD testing for all women aged 65 and older, regardless of additional risk factors.

Reprinted with permission from Physicians' Guide to Prevention and Treatment of Osteoporosis. Washington, DC: National Osteoporosis Foundation; 1999. National Osteoporosis Foundation, Washington, DC 20037.

- **Lifestyle issues** – Important issues for people with or at risk of developing osteoporosis are shown.

Lifestyle Issues Important for Prevention and Treatment of Osteoporosis

Calcium:

Recommended intake is 1,200 mg daily for adults older than 50 years
Most women need a calcium supplement of 500–700 mg daily
Calcium carbonate is effective and least expensive
Calcium citrate often is tolerated better by patients who have digestive distress

Vitamin D:

Recommended intake is 400–800 IU daily
Standard multivitamins contain 400 IU vitamin D
Additional vitamin D (total, 800 IU daily) is advisable for persons older than
 70 years and can be achieved by taking calcium and vitamin D in combination,
 in addition to a multivitamin

Exercise:

Weight-bearing exercise, if possible; recommend walking at least 40 minutes per
 session, at least four sessions per week
Spinal strengthening exercises also are advisable

Avoid cigarette smoking and other possible negative factors, such as high intake of
 caffeine, protein, and phosphorus

Reduce risk of falling

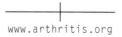

- **Pharmacologic agents** – Medications can reduce the risk of osteoporotic fractures in women who already have had a fracture and in women who have low BMD. Agents approved by the FDA are shown.

FDA-Approved Pharmacologic Agents for Postmenopausal Osteoporosis

Bisphosphonates
Alendronate (Fosamax)
Risedronate (Actonel)
Calcitonin (Miacalcin)[a]
Estrogen (several oral and transdermal preparations)[b]
Raloxifene (Evista)
Teriparatide injection (Forteo)

[a] Calcitonin is approved only for treatment of established osteoporosis.
[b] Estrogen is approved only for prevention of bone loss in recently menopausal women.

- **Bisphosphonates** – Bisphosphonates reduce the ability of individual osteoclasts to resorb bone, reduce the total number of osteoclasts, and accelerate osteoclast apoptosis. They are remarkably free from systemic toxicity.

- **Calcitonin** – Calcitonin acts directly on osteoclasts to reduce bone resorption by binding to specific osteoclast receptors. Nasal calcitonin is extremely well tolerated.

- **Estrogen** – Estrogen is an effective agent for preventing bone loss in recently menopausal women.

- **Raloxifene** – A selective estrogen-receptor modulator (SERM), raloxifene is approved by the FDA for prevention of bone loss in recently menopausal women and for treatment of established osteoporosis.

- **Teriparatide injection** – The first in a new class of drugs called bone formation agents that work primarily to stimulate new bone by increasing the number and action of osteoblasts. Teriparatide is approved for the treatment of osteoporosis in postmenopausal women who are at high risk for a fracture.

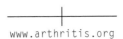

32 THERAPEUTIC INJECTIONS

The major objectives of local injection of joints or soft tissues are to remove fluid and/or to instill therapeutic agents, such as glucocorticoids or hyaluronate, to provide relief of pain.

Indications for Therapeutic Injection of Musculoskeletal Structures

1. When only one or a few joints are inflamed, provided infection has been excluded.

2. In systemic polyarthritis syndromes (e.g. rheumatoid arthritis, psoriatic arthritis, others), as an adjunct to systemic drug therapy.

3. To assist in rehabilitation and prevent deformity.

4. To relieve pain in osteoarthritis exhibiting local inflammatory signs.

5. Soft-tissue regional disorders (e.g. bursitis, tenosynovitis, periarthritis, nodules, epicondylitis, ganglia).

Injection Technique

- **Familiarize** – Successful injection depends on familiarity with the regional anatomy of the structure to be entered.

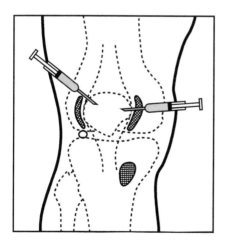

Aspiration and injection sites for the painful knee. The circle lateral to the patellar tendon at the joint line can be entered to deliver glucocorticoids into a flexed knee. Hatched areas on either side of the patella correspond to soft-tissue injection sites. The hatched area medial and inferior to the joint line represents the region of pes anserine bursa.

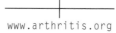

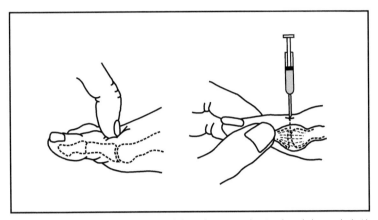

Arthrocentesis/injection of the first metatarsophalangeal joint. Joint line is palpated, then marked with imprint of thumbnail (left panel). Gentle distraction of the phalanx widens joint space, easing entry into capsule by needle oriented perpendicularly to phalanx, penetrating skin at marked joint line just medial to extensor tendon (right panel).

- **Position the patient** – Structures on either side of the injection target should be relaxed.

- **Aseptic injection site** – Skin-cleaning and hand-washing provide sufficient asepsis.

- **Numb injection site** – Spray the site with ethyl chloride solution or infiltrate the skin and subcutaneous tissues with 1% lidocaine.

- **Aspirate** – Evacuating all synovial fluid that can be easily removed minimizes dilution of the injected compound and prolongs relief.

- **Choose glucocorticoid** – Many glucocorticoid preparations are available; less soluble compounds (triamcinolone hexacetonide) are preferred for joint-space injections and provide longer relief.

- **Deliver glucocorticoid** – 1–2 ml of glucocorticoid preparation to large joints (knees, hips, shoulders), half that amount to medium joints (wrists, elbows, ankles), and half again as much (or less) to small joints and soft-tissue sites.

- **Viscosupplementation** – The intra-articular injection of hyaluronan or its derivatives into the knee with OA may reduce pain for up to one year.

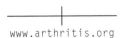

Glucocorticoid Preparations for Therapeutic Injection

Compound (in order of relative solubility)	Concentration (mg/ml)	Glucocorticoid potency (hydrocortisone equivalents/mg)
Triamcinolone hexacetonide[a]	20	5
Triamcinolone acetonide[a]	40	5
Prednisolone tebutate	20	4
Methylprednisolone acetate	20, 40, 80	5
Dexamethasone acetate[a]	8	5
Hydrocortisone acetate	25, 50	1
Triamcinolone diacetate[a]	40	5
Betamethasone sodium phosphate and acetate[a]	6	25
Dexamethasone sodium phosphate	4	25
Prednisolone sodium phosphate	20	4

[a] Fluorinated compounds.

- **Keep a log** – A log in the outpatient record that tracks injections can show overreliance on intra-articular therapy. Joints should not be injected more than 3–4 times a year.

- **Rest joint** – Limiting use of joint for 24 hours after the injection can prolong benefit.

Injections in Specific Disorders

Rheumatoid Arthritis

- **Inflamed, painful joints** – Injections beneficial in acute or chronically inflamed joints. Important to rule out infection before injection.

- **Extra-articular injections** – Certain extra-articular features of RA respond well to local injections, particularly entrapment neuropathies due to synovial proliferation at the volar aspect of the wrist (e.g. carpal tunnel, median nerve), medial aspect of the elbow (cubital tunnel, ulnar nerve), and medial aspect of the ankle (tarsal tunnel, posterior tibial nerve).

Osteoarthritis

- **Controversy** – Widely used, particularly for OA of the knee, but benefit and effects on long-term outcome remain controversial.

- **Pain** – Often arises from structures that are exterior to the joint capsule, and don't respond to intra-articular injections.

Crystalline Arthropathy

- **Diagnosis and treatment** – Joint entry is important for diagnosis of crystalline arthropathy and can be used for treatment often at the same time.

33 NONSTEROIDAL ANTI-INFLAMMATORY DRUGS

Nonsteroidal anti-inflammatory drugs (NSAIDs) have anti-inflammatory, analgesic, and antipyretic properties and are used to reduce pain and inflammation and improve function in people with most forms of arthritis and related diseases. There are at least 20 different NSAIDs currently available in the United States. In addition, cyclooxygenase-2 (COX-2)-specific inhibitors are available with similar efficacy but decreased gastrointestinal (GI) and platelet effects.

Adverse Effects

- **Organ affected** – The NSAIDs may produce toxic effects in several organ systems.

- **GI tract** – The most clinically significant adverse effects occur in the GI tract. Risk factors for developing GI toxicity in people receiving NSAIDs are shown. The approach to the patient who requires chronic NSAID treatment and has developed or is at risk for an NSAID-induced GI event is controversial.

Risk Factors for NSAID-Induced Gastroduodenal Toxic Effects

Increasing patient age (>60 years)
Extent of current and past disease
History of peptic ulcer disease
History of gastrointestinal bleeding
Concomitant use of NSAIDs with glucocorticoid therapy
Dose of the NSAID
Combinations of NSAIDs
History of GI intolerance to NSAIDs

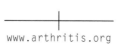

Nonsteroidal Anti-inflammatory Drugs

Drug	Brand name(s)
Diclofenac potassium	Cataflam
Diclofenac sodium	Voltaren Voltaren XR
Diclofenac sodium with misoprostol	Arthrotec
Diflunisal	Dolobid
Etodolac	Lodine Lodine XL
Fenoprofen calcium	Nalfon
Flurbiprofen	Ansaid
Ibuprofen	Prescription: Motrin Non-prescription: Advil, Motrin IB, Nuprin
Indomethacin	Indocin Indocin SR
Ketoprofen	Prescription: Orudis Oruvail Non-prescription: Actron, Orudis KT
Meclofenamate sodium	Meclomen
Mefenamic acid	Ponstel
Meloxicam	Mobic
Nabumetone	Relafen
Naproxen	Naprosyn Naprelan
Naproxen sodium	Prescription: Anaprox Non-prescription: Aleve

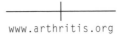

Dosage	Possible side effects
100 to 200 mg per day in 2 or 4 doses	**For all NSAIDs:** Abdominal or stomach cramps, pain or discomfort; edema (swelling of the feet); diarrhea; dizziness; drowsiness or lightheadedness; headache; heartburn or indigestion; nausea or vomiting
100 to 200 mg per day in 2 or 4 doses	
100 mg per day in a single dose	
150 to 200 mg per day in 2 to 4 doses	
500 to 1,500 mg per day in 2 doses	
800 to 1,200 mg per day in 2 to 4 doses	**For diclofenac sodium with misoprostol only:** Same as other NSAIDs except risk of gastric ulcers is decreased; risk of abdominal pain and diarrhea is increased
400 to 1,000 mg per day in a single dose	
900 to 2,400 mg per day in 3 to 4 doses; never more than 3,200 mg per day	
200 to 300 mg per day in 2 to 4 doses	
1,200 to 3,200 mg per day in 3 to 4 doses	
200 to 400 mg every 4 to 6 hours as needed; no more than 3,200 mg per day	
50 to 200 mg in 2 to 4 doses	
75 mg per day in a single dose or 150 mg per day in 2 doses	
200 to 225 mg per day in 3 or 4 doses	
150 to 200 mg per day in a single dose	
12.5 mg every 4 to 6 hours as needed	
200 to 400 mg per day in 4 doses	
250 mg every 6 hours as needed, for up to 7 days	
7.5 to 15 mg per day in a single dose	
1,000 mg per day in 1 or 2 doses; 2,000 mg per day in 2 doses	
500 to 1,500 mg per day in a single dose	
750 mg or 1,000 mg per day in a single dose	
550 to 1,650 mg per day in 2 doses	
220 mg every 8 to 12 hours as needed	

Drug	Brand name(s)
Oxaprozin	Daypro
Piroxicam	Feldene
Sulindac	Clinoril
Tolmetin sodium	Tolectin
COX-2 inhibitors	
Celecoxib	Celebrex
Salicylates	
Acetylated salicylates	
Aspirin	Non-prescription: Anacin, Ascriptin, Bayer, Bufferin, Ecotrin, Excedrin tablets
Nonacetylated salicylates	
Choline and magnesium salicylates	CMT, Tricosal, Trilisate
Choline salicylate	Arthropan
Magnesium salicylate	Prescription: Magan, Mobidin, Mobogesic Non-prescription: Arthritab, Bayer Select, Doan's Pills
Salsalate	Amigesic, Analfex 750, Disalcid, Marthritic, MonoGesic, Salflex, Salsitab
Sodium salicylate	(Available as generic only)

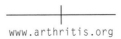

www.arthritis.org

Dosage	Possible side effects
1,200 to 1,800 mg per day in a single dose	**For all NSAIDs:** Abdominal or stomach cramps, pain or discomfort; edema (swelling of the feet); diarrhea; dizziness; drowsiness or lightheadedness; headache; heartburn or indigestion; nausea or vomiting
20 mg per day in 1 or 2 doses	
300 to 400 mg per day in 2 doses	
1,200 to 1,800 mg per day in 3 doses	
200 mg per day in 1 or 2 doses or 400 mg per day in 2 doses	**For Celebrex:** Same as traditional NSAIDs, except less likely to cause bleeding stomach ulcers and susceptibility to bruising and bleeding
2,400 to 5,400 mg per day in several doses	**For all salicylates:** Abdominal or stomach cramps, pain, or discomfort; edema (swelling of the feet); diarrhea; dizziness; drowsiness or lightheadedness; headache; heartburn or indigestion; nausea or vomiting
2,000 to 3,000 mg per day in 2 or 3 doses	
3,480 mg or 20 ml per day in several doses	
2,600 to 4,800 mg per day in 3 to 6 doses	
1,000 to 3,000 mg per day in 2 or 3 doses	
3,600 to 5,400 mg per day in several doses	

- **Kidney** – The effects of NSAIDs on renal function include sodium retention, changes in tubular function, interstitial nephritis, and reversible renal failure due to alterations in filtration rate and renal plasma flow. Risk factors for renal failure associated with NSAID use are shown.

- **Liver** – Elevations of transaminases (SGOT and SGPT) are common, but generally not clinically important. Rare cases of hepatic failure have been noted with all NSAIDs.

- **CNS** – Wide variety of CNS symptoms possible including headaches, confusion, depression, vertigo, tremors, and aseptic meningitis.

Prophylaxis and Treatment of NSAID-Induced GI Disease

Antacids
No data demonstrate usefulness
Sucralfate
No data demonstrate prevention or improvement of gastric ulcers
H2-antagonists
Heal duodenal lesions Prevent duodenal lesions High dosages prevent gastric lesions and heal NSAID-induced lesions Improve symptoms
Omeprazole
Demonstrates prophylaxis and heals both gastroduodenal lesions Improves symptoms
Misoprostol
Heals NSAID-induced gastroduodenal erosive disease 200 mg q.i.d. prevents NSAID-induced gastric and duodenal disease 200 mg b.i.d., t.i.d., q.i.d. prevents NSAID-induced erosive disease Does not improve symptoms

b.i.d., twice per day; t.i.d., three times per day; q.i.d., four times per day.

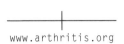

www.arthritis.org

Risk Factors for Renal Failure Associated with NSAIDs

High risk
Volume depletion, such as hemodynamically significant bleed, or a patient with hemodynamic compromise, such as septic shock Severe congestive heart failure Hepatic cirrhosis with or without ascites Clinically significant dehydration
Low to moderate risk
Intrinsic renal disease 　　Diabetic nephropathy 　　Nephrotic syndrome 　　Hypertensive nephropathy Induction of anesthesia
Questionable risk
Advanced age

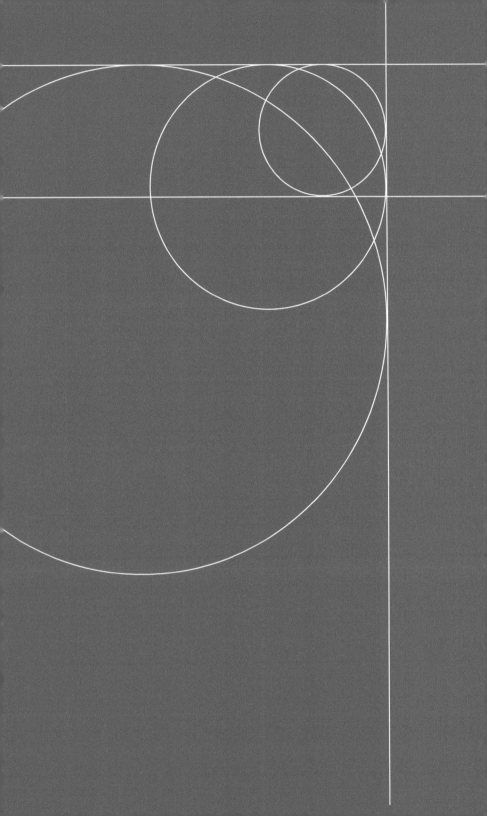

34 GLUCOCORTICOIDS

Glucocorticoids are powerful anti-inflammatory and immunomodulatory drugs that are effective in the management of many rheumatic diseases.

Mechanism of Action

- **Immune cells** – Glucocorticoids act through a wide variety of mechanisms. These include: inhibition of leukocyte trafficking and access to sites of inflammation; disruption of the functions of leukocytes, fibroblasts, and endothelial cells; and suppression of the production and actions of humoral factors involved in the inflammatory process. The important effects glucocorticoids have on immune cells are shown in the following table.

Anti-inflammatory Effects of Glucocorticoids on Immune Cells

Cells affected	Effect of glucocorticoid
Monocytes/ macrophages	↓ number of circulating cells (↓ myelopoiesis, ↓ release) ↓ expression of MHC class II molecules and Fc receptors ↓ synthesis of pro-inflammatory cytokines (e.g. IL2, IL6, TNFα) and prostaglandins
T cells	↓ number of circulating cells (redistribution effects) ↓ production and action of IL2 (most important)
Granulocytes	↓ number of eosinophils and basophils ↑ number of circulating neutrophils (through demargination)
Endothelial cells	↓ vessel permeability ↓ expression of adhesion molecules ↓ production of IL1 and prostaglandins
Fibroblasts	↓ proliferation ↓ production of fibronectin

Fc, crystallizable fragment of immunoglobulin; IL, interleukin; MHC, major histocompatibility complex; TNF, tumor necrosis factor.
Reproduced from Buttgereit F, et al. The molecular basis for the effectiveness, toxicity, and resistance to glucocorticoids: focus on the treatment of rheumatoid arthritis. Scand J Rheum 2005; 34: 14–21. Reprinted with permission of Taylor & Francis Ltd.

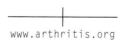

Glucocorticoid Doses and their Clinical Use

Terminology	Dosage (mg/day equivalent of prednisolone)	Clinical application
Low dose	≤7.5	Maintenance therapy for rheumatic disease
Medium dose	>7.5 to ≤30	Initial therapy for primary chronic rheumatic disease
High dose	>30 to ≤100	Initial therapy for subacute rheumatic disease
Very high dose	>100	Initial therapy for acute and/or life-threatening exacerbations of rheumatic diseases
Pulse therapy	≥250 for one to a few days	For severe and/or life-threatening exacerbations of rheumatic diseases

- **Genomic mechanisms** – Cytosolic glucocorticoid receptor (cGCR)-mediated effects refer to the up- or downregulation of specific regulatory proteins. The activated glucocorticoid/cGCR complex binds to specific DNA-binding sites called glucocorticoid responsive elements. The subsequent upregulation of certain proteins is termed transactivation. Transrepression is a key aspect of the mode of action of glucocorticoids.

- **Transrepression** – Refers to the inhibition of the glucocorticoid/cGCR complex mediated by NF-κB and activator protein-1. This results in the downregulation of pro-inflammatory cytokines such as IL1, IL6, and TNFα, and of prostaglandins.

- **Nongenomic mechanisms** – cGCR-mediated nongenomic effects may occur alongside the genomic effects, whereby ligand binding initiates a rapid release of proteins (chaperones and co-chaperones) from the multiprotein complex. Glucocorticoids also mediate rapid and therapeutic effects via membrane-bound GCR. In addition, high levels of glucocorticoids may interact with cellular membranes and alter their properties.

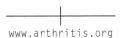

Adverse effects
Relatively few
Dose-dependent and considerable in longer-term use
Not suitable for long-term therapy because of severe adverse effects
Not suitable for long-term therapy because of severe, dramatic adverse effects
High proportion of cases with relatively low incidence of adverse effects

Clinical Use

● **Anti-inflammatory effects** – Occur mostly through transrepression.

● **Inhibition of radiological progression** – By reducing the synthesis of IL1 and TNFα, glucocorticoids disrupt the effects of these on osteoclasts which are responsible for bone resorption/erosion.

● **Daily practice** – Standardized glucocorticoid dosing is shown in the table.

● **Glucocorticoid resistance** – Several mechanisms are implicated in glucocorticoid resistance:

- reduced number of GCRs and/or reduced affinity of the ligand

- polymorphic changes and/or overexpression of chaperones/co-chaperones

- increased expression of inflammatory transcription factors

- changes in the phosphorylation status of the GCR

- overexpression of GCR-β

- multidrug resistance gene (MDR1)

- alteration in the expression of membrane-bound GCRs.

Adverse Events

● **Musculoskeletal** – Osteoporosis, osteonecrosis, and proximal myopathy.

● **Endocrine and metabolic** – Redistribution of body fat and weight gain with chronic glucocorticoid use. Patients at risk for diabetes are also at risk of developing new-onset hyperglycemia during glucocorticoid use.

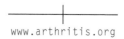

- **Cardiovascular (CV)** – Glucocorticoids induce dyslipidemia and prolonged administration contributes to CV disease. Hypertension is observed in ~20% of patients receiving glucocorticoids. Rare CV events include arrhythmias and sudden death, but these appear to occur only with high-dose pulse therapy.

- **Dermatologic** – Cushingoid appearance and ease of bruising are common effects of chronic glucocorticoid use.

- **Ophthalmologic** – Cataracts, glaucoma.

- **Gastrointestinal (GI)** – Possible increased risk of GI ulcers, particularly if used in combination with nonsteroidal anti-inflammatory drugs.

- **Infectious** – Increased susceptibility to various viral, bacterial, fungal, and parasitic infections.

- **Psychological and behavioral** – Minor or major mood disturbances or psychoses.

New Developments

- **Liposomes** – For targeted delivery of glucocorticoids.

- **Timed-release formulation** – To improve the timing of the delivery of glucocorticoids.

- **Glycyrrhetinic acid** – Inhibits 11-β-hydroxysteroid dehydrogenase and increases levels of endogenous glucocorticoid.

- **Nitrosteroids** – Aliphatic or aromatic molecules that link a glucocorticoid drug with nitric oxide. The nitric oxide that is slowly released and the attached glucocorticoid appear to have synergistic anti-inflammatory effects.

- **Selective glucocorticoid receptor agonists (SEGRAs)** – Also known as dissociating glucocorticoids. SEGRAs act predominantly via the preferred transrepression mechanism rather than by transactivation, which can be associated with adverse effects such as diabetes and glaucoma.

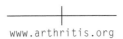

35 OPERATIVE TREATMENT

Surgical interventions play an important role in the management of pain that is unresponsive to conventional treatment, and in improving joint function that has been impaired by arthritis. A wide variety of surgical options for the management of arthritis are available.

Operative Treatments

Joint debridement

Synovectomy

Osteotomy

Soft-tissue arthroplasty

Resection arthroplasty

Fusion

Joint replacement

Tenosynovectomy

Repair of reconstruction of ruptured tendons

Hip

- **Arthroplasty** – Joint replacement (total joint arthroplasty) is the most commonly used and successful operative treatment for arthritis of the hip, particularly in patients with end-stage osteoarthritis (OA) or rheumatoid arthritis (RA). Prostheses may be cemented (i.e. anchored with polymethylmethacrylate cement) or uncemented (bone growth directly into the prosthesis). This is a highly successful method of treating pain and disability.

- **Osteotomies and fusions** – Performed less frequently than hip replacements, but can produce good results in certain patients.

Knee

- **Synovectomy** – Synovectomy, typically by arthroscopy, can decrease pain and swelling in patients with RA unresponsive to other treatments, or with rare forms of arthritis, such as hemophilia, pigmented villonodular synovitis, and synovial chondromatosis.

- **Arthroscopic debridement or chondroplasty** – May provide short-term relief of symptoms in OA.

- **Osteotomy** – Used in OA to redirect weight-bearing away from the tibiofemoral joint. Osteotomies are often chosen over total knee arthroplasties for young, overweight, active patients.

- **Arthroplasty** – Total joint replacement is highly effective at relieving pain and improving function, particularly in OA and RA (and related inflammatory forms of arthritis).

- **Arthrodesis (fusion)** – A consideration in patients with recalcitrant infection or failed total knee arthroplasty that cannot be revised effectively.

Foot and Ankle

- **Cheilectomy** – Cheilectomy (resection of an osteophyte) often provides relief of symptoms in patients with OA affecting the feet, most commonly performed for treatment of hallux valgus (a bunion).

- **Osteotomy** – May be used in OA to realign joints and relieve the pain of weight-bearing joints.

- **Arthrodesis** – Arthrodesis provides pain relief and stability; used in patients with severe, destructive arthritis.

Hand and Wrist

- **Ruptured tendons** – Inability to actively flex or extend interphalangeal and/or metacarpophalangeal joints, with preservation of passive motion, usually signals a ruptured tendon. Acute tendon ruptures should be evaluated early for consideration of reconstruction.

- **Digit drift** – Ulnar drift of the digits commonly occurs in RA as a result of subluxation of the extensor tendons. This may be corrected by surgical repositioning of the tendon and transferring the intrinsic muscle insertions.

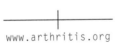

- **Tenosynovectomy** – Inflammation of tendon sheaths within the palm are a frequent problem in RA and other inflammatory arthropathies. Tenosynovectomy decreases pain, increases range of motion and grip strength, and protects the tendons from rupture.

- **Joint reconstruction** – Metacarpophalangeal joints of the fingers may be reconstructed with silicone implants (Swanson implants) that function as flexible spacers. The procedure is commonly used in RA associated with advanced deformities that impair hand function.

- **Arthrodesis** – May be used in interphalangeal joints (most commonly the thumb) or the wrist to stabilize the joint and improve hand function.

Elbow

- **Radial-head resection** – Allows for increased range of motion and decreased pain; useful in appropriately selected patients with advanced, destructive arthritis of the elbow.

- **Synovectomy** – May be performed alone or in conjunction with other procedures, such as radial-head resection, in patients with chronic inflammatory synovitis of the elbow unresponsive to other therapies.

- **Arthroplasty** – Elbow joint replacement has developed rapidly, and is a reasonable consideration in people with advanced destructive arthritis.

Shoulder

- **Arthroplasty** – Effective for relief of pain and improvement of function in glenohumeral arthritis.

Cervical Spine

- **Spinal fusions** – Can decrease pain, restore stability and, in some instances, prevent development of neurologic deficits.

- **Surgical decompression** – Spinal cord and nerve root decompression can relieve pain and improve neurologic function.

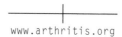

- **Arthrodesis** – Patients who undergo cervical arthrodesis earlier in the course of their disease have more satisfactory results than those in whom arthrodesis is delayed.

- **Posterior decompression** – May be accomplished via laminectomy or laminaplasty.

36 COMPLEMENTARY AND ALTERNATIVE THERAPIES

Complementary and alternative medicines (CAM) are widely used by people with arthritis and related diseases. It is important that healthcare providers are familiar with the most commonly used CAM therapies to respond to queries from patients. Questions regarding the use of CAM therapies should be asked as a part of the comprehensive history and physical examination.

The most popular and commonly used CAM therapies include:

- **Meditation, biofeedback, and stress reduction** – Used widely for the treatment of pain, depression, and anxiety. These therapeutic modalities are particularly popular with people who have fibromyalgia.

- **Exercise** – Strengthening, stretching, general conditioning exercises, and yoga have been shown to provide symptomatic relief for various forms of arthritis.

- **Acupuncture** – Used to treat pain in diverse conditions, such as osteoarthritis, fibromyalgia, and low back pain.

- **Herbs, supplements, and vitamins** – Widely used for osteoarthritis, fibromyalgia, and nonspecific musculoskeletal pain. Potential for harmful side effects or interactions with prescription medications.

  - **Dehydroepiandrosterone (DHEA)** – An androgen steroid hormone naturally produced in the body. Levels of DHEA are low in people with RA and lupus. Studies show that when used in conjunction with conventional lupus treatment, DHEA may reduce disease flares.

  - **Fish oil** – Oil from cold-water fish contains omega-3 fatty acids. Studies show that fish supplements, alone and in combination with conventional drugs, are effective in treating RA symptoms.

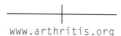

— **Glucosamine** – Provides building blocks for growth, repair, and maintenance of cartilage. Studies show that glucosamine eases OA symptoms and may slow the progression of the disease and reduce cartilage loss.

— **Chondroitin** – A component of cartilage, bone, and tendon. Studies show that chondroitin improves pain, inflammation, and joint function.

— **SAM-e** – An effective anti-inflammatory and analgesic for people with OA.

— **Vitamin C** – Necessary for collagen formation and tissue repair. Studies show vitamin C decreases OA pain and risk of progression.

— **Vitamin D** – Builds bone mass, prevents bone loss and muscle weakness, aids in calcium absorption, and may slow OA progression.

INDEX

A

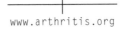

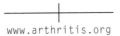

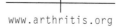

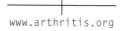

www.arthritis.org